Evidence-based Audit in General Practice
From principles to practice

Edited by

Robin C. Fraser MD, FRCGP
Professor of General Practice

Mayur K. Lakhani MRCGP, MRCP
Lecturer in Clinical Audit

Richard H. Baker MD, FRCGP
Director

Eli Lilly National Clinical Audit Centre,
Department of General Practice and Primary Health Care,
University of Leicester, UK

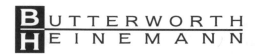
BUTTERWORTH
HEINEMANN

OXFORD   BOSTON   JOHANNESBURG   MELBOURNE   NEW DELHI   SINGAPORE

Butterworth-Heinemann
Linacre House, Jordan Hill, Oxford OX2 8DP
225 Wildwood Avenue, Woburn, MA 01801-2041
A division of Reed Educational and Professional Publishing Ltd

℞ A member of the Reed Elsevier plc group

First published 1998
Reprinted 1999

British Library Cataloguing in Publication Data
A catalogue record for this book is available from the British Library

Library of Congress Cataloguing in Publication Data
A catalogue record for this book is available from the Library of Congress

ISBN 0 7506 3104 X

Typeset by Keyword Typesetting Services Ltd

Printed and bound in Great Britain by Biddles Ltd, Guildford and King's Lynn

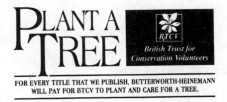

FOR EVERY TITLE THAT WE PUBLISH, BUTTERWORTH-HEINEMANN
WILL PAY FOR BTCV TO PLANT AND CARE FOR A TREE.

Evidence-based Audit in General Practice

HIG4

Contents

Contributors

Richard Baker MD (London) FRCGP
Director, Eli Lilly National Clinical Audit Centre, Department of General Practice and Primary Health Care, University of Leicester

Tim Coleman MB ChB (Leeds) MRCGP
Clinical Lecturer, Department of General Practice and Primary Health Care, University of Leicester; General Practitioner, Leicester

Azhar Farooqi MB ChB (Manchester) FRCGP DCH DRCOG
Chair, Leicestershire Primary Care Audit Group, Leicestershire Health Authority; General Practitioner, Leicester

Robin Fraser MD (Aberdeen) FRCGP
Professor of General Practice and Head, Department of General Practice and Primary Health Care, University of Leicester; General Practitioner, Leicester

Kamlesh Khunti MB ChB (Dundee) FRCGP DCH DRCOG
Lecturer in Clinical Audit, Eli Lilly National Clinical Audit Centre, Department of General Practice and Primary Health Care, University of Leicester; General Practitioner, Leicester

Mayur Lakhani MB ChB (Dundee) MRCP MRCGP DCH
Lecturer in Clinical Audit, Eli Lilly National Clinical Audit Centre, Department of General Practice and Primary Health Care, University of Leicester; General Practitioner, Loughborough

Rosalind Sorrie BSc (Aberdeen) MSc (Leicester Polytechnic)
Manager, Primary Care Audit Group, Leicestershire Health Authority

Foreword

The principal of clinical audit is not new. Thoughtful and conscientious clinicians have long been used to collecting series of similar cases, analysing their results, digesting the significance of these, and modifying their practice where appropriate to do so. Clinical audit as we know it took shape in general practice in the 1970s, when some general practices saw the value of clinical enquiry and self scrutiny, and the benefits to practice of peer-driven external comparison and review.

However, despite determined efforts by the RCGP in the 1980s to extend this habit of self-scrutiny to all general practices, inertia within the wider profession was too entrenched and powerful to overcome from within. The results we all know. Mrs Thatcher's government, as part of its health reforms, took matters into his own hands by setting up an infrastructure for clinical audit within general practice (the Medical Audit Advisory Groups) and by making audit a contractual responsibility for consultants. The current government, with its plans for a National Institute of Clinical Excellence, a Commission on Health Improvement, and strengthened accountability through local clinical governance, places even more priority on quality. The object, around which both the profession and government can unite, is to try and secure improvement in the quality of patient care, reduce variations in the performance of doctors which cannot be justified, and eliminate poor practice since it constitutes a potential hazard to patients.

This is a fast moving agenda. Today the profession is becoming accustomed to working with explicit standards, and to monitoring performance against these. There is a growth industry in clincal guidelines, and general practice can be proud of the fact that it has produced some of the best of these. In its booklet *Good Medical Practice* the General Medical Council expects all doctors to maintain a good standard of practice by keeping up-to-date, monitoring their own performance through clinical audit, and ensuring their professional development by applying the results of regular appraisal.

Clinical audit is presented, rightly, as a series of opportunities for sustained improvement. Encouragement, rather than threat, is seen as the preferred motivator. Nevertheless, the very use of audit does reveal substandard practice, and will leave substandard practitioners with no hiding place. It is as well that audit is now becoming established as an integral and fundamental part of medical practice, for the public expectation of doctors is rising, public awareness of what is and is not acceptable practice is becoming more widespread, and public intolerance of poor practice is becoming more determined.

In their book Professor Robin Fraser and his colleagues make a valuable contribution to this unfolding agenda. Like several other manuals available today, they describe what audit is in general practice and how to do it. But, importantly, they then move on. They link audit explicity to the evidence-base for good general practice, and demonstrate very lucidly how the principles of evidence-based clinical audit can be applied in important areas of care in general practice by giving a series of detailed examples.

Readers will find the book accessible and easily readable, with material which will be readily translatable into any general practice in the United Kingdom.

Donald Irvine

Preface

> Participation in audit is probably the most effective way of enabling GPs and primary health care teams to monitor and improve the quality of care they deliver to their patients.

It is many years since general practitioners (GPs) were first encouraged to make (clinical) audit 'an integral part of their day to day activities' (Irvine, 1983). Recently, the General Medical Council (GMC) decreed that it was the duty of every doctor 'to monitor and improve the quality of health care' and 'to take part in regular and systematic clinical audit' (GMC, 1995). Successive governments have also placed clinical audit and quality high on their respective agendas for the NHS (Department of Health, 1989 and 1997). Meanwhile, evidence was accumulating that participation in systematic audit could bring about substantial improvements in patient care. Indeed, 'It could be argued that clinical audit can be the central and most useful tool for improving quality and/or cost-effectiveness of patient care in the NHS' (Fraser and Baker, 1997).

Although levels of participation in clinical audit by GPs was impressive – by 1994, 90 per cent of practices were undertaking some form of audit (Baker et al., 1995) – it was becoming clear that many practices were encountering difficulties in the practical implementation of audit. Many audits were not 'completing the cycle' and others were based on criteria which were not chosen systematically. As a consequence, improvements in care were often disappointing in relation to the expenditure of effort by the involved practice personnel. Furthermore, despite the fact that audit was a criterion for recognition as a training practice, it was discovered that '. . . experienced GP trainers are struggling to recognize even basic audit methodology' (Lough and Murray, 1997). Moreover, many trainers were found to be '. . . unaware of this deficiency. . .'. It was concluded that 'considerable help needs to be given to overcome this' (Lough and Murray, 1997).

The main purpose of this book is to familiarize GPs, and other members of the practice team, with the principles of systematic clinical audit and to indicate how these can be applied to the day to day work of general practices. By so doing, it is our hope that the book can assist and encourage practices to undertake audit which is underpinned by evidence-based and prioritized audit criteria. If followed, this approach is highly likely to promote behavioural change which will influence quality of care for the better. Thus, the book should help practices interested in undertaking audit to concentrate their efforts on audit activities which will maximize returns on their investment of professional time. It should also help training practices to improve standards of teaching of audit methodologies.

Readers should be clear, therefore, that throughout this book we shall be referring to audit which is both professionally led and undertaken voluntarily by GPs and practice teams (in both training and non-training practices) for professional development and quality improvement purposes.

The book naturally divides into two interlinked parts. The first three chapters cover the principles and historical development of audit in general practice, outline a generic approach to the development of evidence-based and prioritized audit criteria and detail practical steps which should be followed in undertaking any audit. This removes the need to duplicate detailed descriptions of the process of developing audit criteria and the practical steps in undertaking the five specimen audits presented in Chapters 4–8. We have selected the topics to confirm that the approach to audit which we are advocating can be applied 'across the board' to any clinical or organizational field in general practice. To further minimize the need for practices to 'reinvent the wheel' we have also included specimen audit recording forms which can be (photo)copied as required.

In Appendix 1 we list all the currently available audit protocols developed by the Lilly Audit Centre and reproduce the 'must do' criteria from these protocols. As an *aide-mémoire* to practices we also include, in Appendix 2, a check-list to assist a practice in monitoring (and amending as necessary) the steps it needs to take in preparing for, carrying out and reviewing any audit project it undertakes.

We hope that you will find this book useful in your audit endeavours – remember taking part in audit can be both stimulating and enjoyable. Finally we would be pleased to receive feedback from readers on any aspect of the book – please write to us or e-mail us at clinaudit@le.ac.uk.

Robin Fraser
Mayur Lakhani
Richard Baker

References

Baker, R., Hearnshaw, H., Robertson, N. *et al.* (1995) Assessing the work of medical audit advisory groups in promoting audit in general practice. *Quality in Health Care* **4**: 234–239.

Department of Health (1989) Working for patients. Working Paper No. 6. London: Department of Health.

Department of Health (1997) The new NHS (Cm 3807). London: Department of Health.

Fraser, R.C. and Baker, R. (1997) The clinical audit programme in England: achievements and challenges. *Audit Trends* **5**: 131–136.

General Medical Council (1995) Good medical practice. London: GMC.

Irvine, D.H. (1983) Quality of care in general practice: our outstanding problem. *J. Roy. Coll. Gen Pract.* **33**: 521–523.

Lough, J.R.M. and Murray, S. (1997) Training for audit: Lessons still to be learned. *Br. J. Gen. Pract.* **47**: 743–746.

Acknowledgements

The editors would like to acknowledge the assistance given by the following people in the preparation of this book: Helen Foster, Vicki Cluley and Hilary Bracey for cheerfully typing a succession of drafts; departmental colleagues for their comments and suggestions; the editors of the *British Journal of General Practice* and *Primary Care Psychiatry* for permission to quote work (in Chapters 2 and 8 respectively); and Mary Seager and Hannah Tudge and the staff of Butterworth-Heinemann for their encouragement and professional support. Last but not least, we are most grateful to Sir Donald Irvine for agreeing to write the Foreword; this is particularly fitting since Sir Donald was the prime mover of the quality initiative in general practice and he has continued to make a major contribution in this area.

Evidence-based clinical audit: an overview

Introduction

Many general practitioners (GPs) and practice team members have been involved in medical audit to a varying extent for many years. Nevertheless, there is still some uncertainty about what medical audit is, how it should best be implemented in practice and the extent to which involvement in audit can facilitate improvements in the delivery or outcome of patient care. Accordingly, in this chapter, we will provide an explicit definition of audit, advise on a systematic and proven approach to its practical implementation and provide some evidence of the value of participation in audit. We shall also trace the historical milestones in the development of medical audit in general practice, describe the change in focus from medical to clinical audit and emphasize the need for the incorporation of research evidence in any criteria against which actual performance is to be judged.

What is meant by the term 'medical audit'?

In the White Paper that led to the creation of a national structure to support audit throughout the NHS, audit was defined as: 'The systematic, critical analysis of the quality of medical care, including the procedures used for diagnosis and treatment, the use of resources, and the resulting outcome and quality of life for the patient' (Secretaries of State, 1989). Although this definition makes clear that audit can be concerned with almost any aspect of care, and that it should be undertaken systematically, it fails to include any explicit reference to two key components of the audit process. The first is the need for participants in audit to be prepared to make necessary changes in professional behaviour; the second is the requirement to attempt to demonstrate improvements in the quality and/or cost-effectiveness of care delivered as a consequence of participation in audit.

Marinker (1990) subsequently suggested that: 'Medical audit is the attempt to improve quality of medical care by measuring the performance of those providing that care, by considering the performance in relation to desired standards and by improving on this performance'. A similar definition was put forward by Crombie *et al.* (1993): 'Audit is the process of reviewing the delivery of health care to identify deficiencies so that they may be remedied'. These two definitions represent an improvement because they make clear that the purpose of audit is to improve care, but they still place insufficient emphasis on the need to conduct the review of care in a systematic way. An additional problem with all three definitions, however, is that they do not sufficiently reflect the essential *personal* commitment of health professionals to monitor and improve their *own* professional activities which is of critical importance in determining whether audit projects will be completed successfully or not.

Accordingly, we would prefer to recommend the following definition of audit, as it incorporates all the essential conceptual and practical underpinnings of the audit process: 'Audit is the process of critically and systematically assessing our own professional activities with a commitment to improving personal performance and, ultimately, the quality and/or cost-effectiveness of patient care' (Fraser, 1982). This definition also signifies that successful outcomes of involvement in audit can result in improvements in quality *and* cost-effectiveness, or alternatively, that use of resources can be improved while maintaining standards of care.

The evolution of audit in general practice

Contrary to popular belief, audit in general practice is not new, as a number of single practice developments in audit began more than 20 years ago (Crombie *et al.*, 1993). The first major commitment to audit, however, was made by the Royal College of General Practitioners (RCGP) in 1977 in its evidence to the Royal Commission on the NHS. The College acknowledged deficiencies in the quality of UK general practice, and with commendable foresight, recognized the potential influence of medical audit as a means of improving standards of care. Shortly afterwards, this lead was followed by the General Medical Services Committee, a Special Conference of Local Medical Committees and the Fourth National Trainee Conference. Thus, four national bodies representing all shades of general practice opinion – academic, political and future doctors – had endorsed the principle of voluntary participation in audit by all GPs (see Box 1.1).

Box 1.1. Milestones in the development of audit in general practice

• 1977	Royal College of General Practitioners (RCGP)	Called for professionally led audit.
• 1979	General Medical Services Committee	Called for professionally led audit.
• 1979	Special Conference of Local Medical Committees	Called for professionally led audit.
• 1979	Royal Commission on the National Health Service	Called for professionally led audit.
• 1981	Fourth National Trainee Conference	Only 31% of trainees introduced to any form of audit. Called for professionally led audit.
• 1983	RCGP Quality Initiative	Within 10 years all GPs should incorporate standard setting and performance review as an integral part of their professional lives.
• 1991	Medical Audit Advisory Groups	The objective was the participation of all practices by April 1992.
• 1991	Joint Committee of Postgraduate Training for General Practice (JCPTGP)	Audit made a required component of vocational training.
• 1995	General Medical Council	Participation in audit recognized as one of the duties of a doctor.
• 1995	Clinical Outcomes Group Report: Clinical audit in primary health care	Specified how clinical audit care could be developed in primary health care.
• 1996	JCPTGP	Submission of audit project part of (mandatory) summative assessment of vocational training.

Further encouragement – and a call to action – was provided by the Royal Commission on the NHS (1979) which recommended that 'General practitioners should make local arrangements specifically to facilitate audit of the services they provide'. There was also a call for the creation of 'Local Audit Committees' to provide 'Advisory and support services. . . and points of entry for interested doctors' (Fraser, 1981). By 1983, however, there was little sign of co-ordinated activity or mass involvement in audit by GPs when the RCGP launched its famous 'Quality Initiative'. In seeking to stimulate more activity Irvine stated: 'We have talked about improving the quality of care in general practice for long enough. We should now adopt a policy which can turn hopes into reality . . .' (Irvine, 1983). In articulating the need for the Quality Initiative, Irvine also stated there was too great a gap in standards between good and bad general practice. He described the issue of quality of care as 'our outstanding problem' and called on all GPs to incorporate standard setting and systematic performance review as an integral part of their day-to-day work. Between 1983 and 1989 the RCGP continued to recommend audit without much success, the GMSC did not press the issue and audit was regarded less than enthusiastically by GP vocational trainees.

Perhaps irritated at the lack of professional activity, the Government decreed in its 1989 White Paper (Secretaries of State, 1989) that some form of involvement in medical audit would, for the first time, become a contractual responsibility for all GPs. (The contractual requirement was subsequently dropped in favour of voluntary involvement.) In 1991, funds were made available to set up Medical Audit Advisory Groups (MAAGs) for every family health services authority (FHSA) in England and Wales and their equivalents in Scotland and Northern Ireland. The principal remit of the MAAGs was to ensure the participation of all GPs in regular and systematic audit through the provision of appropriate advice and support. Although sub-committees of the FHSAs, MAAGs were to be professionally led and semi-autonomous, and were destined to play a key role in the implementation of audit. Most MAAGs employed lay audit support staff to assist in facilitating audit participation both in individual practice projects and in single topic audits in which all local practices were invited to become involved.

Mainly through the efforts of the MAAGs, the proportion of practices participating in audit rose from 57 per cent in 1991/92 to 86 per cent in 1993/94 (Baker *et al.*, 1995). This represented rapid and substantial progress, since prior to the launch of the national audit programme, there was a very low level of data collection in general practice, let alone participation in audit. For example, in a 1982 survey of 508 practices in Leicestershire and Lincolnshire (which were typical of all practices in England), it was found that only 20 per cent of practices collected *any* data on *any* aspect of practice performance (Fraser and Gosling, 1985). Furthermore, less than 10 per cent of the practices which did collect data used them to change practice procedures or policies.

The wider involvement of GPs in audit was also greatly assisted by the decision taken in 1991 by the Joint Committee of Postgraduate Training for General Practice (JCPTGP) to require training practices to involve vocational trainees in audit. As a direct consequence, all recent entrants to general practice should be familiar with the principles of audit and their practical implementation. This desirable state of affairs was reinforced in 1996 when the JCPTGP decreed that the submission of an audit project would be a required part of (mandatory) summative assessment of vocational training. Henceforth, all new entrants to general practice would have had to *demonstrate* their ability to complete an audit satisfactorily.

The Report on Clinical Audit in Primary Health Care (1995) commented that 'remarkable progress has been made in implementing clinical audit, particularly in general practice, given that there are no contractual obligations to carry out audit and no resources regularly committed to individual practice units for this purpose'. Having praised the role of MAAGs, the report suggested that 'clinical audit facilitation should become part of a wider range of support for quality assurance and development available for practices'. The report also reinforced the importance of audit remaining professionally led and called for a strengthening of 'the linkage of clinical audit with the training and continuing education of all health professionals. . . .'. The report was clear, however, that 'the results of clinical audit should not be used for contract monitoring'.

It seems clear, therefore, that audit is here to stay; indeed it is regarded as the central plank in the clinical effectiveness programme throughout the NHS (NHS Executive 1996a, 1996b).

From 'medical' to 'clinical' audit

From 1990 onwards, the development of audit in the setting of general practice became incorporated in, and was influenced by, the strategic priorities of the national audit programme and their practical consequences. From 1990 to 1994 the priority was to involve *all* health professionals, not just the doctors, in audit . Initially, individual health professionals were encouraged to participate with their colleagues from within the same discipline. Latterly, it was expected that there should be a transition from uniprofessional to multidisciplinary audit, from individual to team involvement and to audit across the interface between primary and secondary care. Gradually, the term 'medical' audit which referred to audit carried out by medical doctors, was replaced by the term 'clinical' audit which referred to audit carried out by health professionals who may include doctors or not. Clinical audit has been defined as: 'The process by which doctors, nurses and other health professionals regularly and systematically review, and where necessary change, their clinical practice' (Primary Health Care Clinical Audit Working Group, 1995).

The transition from medical to clinical audit was a natural step for many GPs, their primary health care teams, and for the MAAGs (Humphrey and Berrow, 1993). Indeed, many MAAGs changed their name to primary care audit groups (PCAGs) to reflect their new role and composition as some medical members were replaced by representatives of practice nurses, practice managers and patient groups. This latter representation reflected the increased involvement in, and the valuable contribution to, audit that 'consumers of health care' could make.

Carrying out audit: a systematic approach

Audit is a cycle or spiral which consists of a series of particular steps (see Box 1.2). At this stage it is our intention to outline only the essential features, as full details of the method will be described in Chapter 3.

Box 1.2   A systematic approach to audit: the essential steps

- Select topic.
- Identify specific aims.
- Agree target criteria and standards.
- Devise method of data collection.
- Collect data.
- Analyse and compare with target criteria and standards.
- Agree and implement changes.
- Collect further data to evaluate change.

An audit project begins with the need to select a topic, followed by the formulation of explicit aims and the identification of explicit criteria, preferably evidence-based and prioritized, against which to judge performance. Actual performance must be determined by the collection of objective data. Discrepancies between actual and desired performance then need to be addressed by selected strategies which may include feedback, facilitation or reminders. Data are then collected again to determine the extent to which appropriate changes have been made. Activities which comply with this systematic and sequential approach are most likely to bring about improvements in care. Activities which do not usually involve aimless data collection which inevitably leads to disillusionment and demotivation of participants as they can see no clear advantage or end point. Underlying deficiencies in design or methodology result in participants expending enormous amounts of energy without any prospect of a successful conclusion.

Topic selection

Since audits can be carried out on a wide variety of clinical and organizational topics, choices of specific audit topics have to be made, preferably by those who are to be involved in the audit. To obtain the best return on the effort involved, potential topics should be compared with the factors outlined in Box 1.3 before a final choice is made.

Box 1.3 Factors to consider when selecting a topic for audit

Factor	Consequence
• Important impact on health.	Likely increase in morbidity/mortality if care is poor.
• Affects a large number of people.	Improving quality of care in common conditions usually has more impact than in rare conditions.
• Convincing evidence is available about appropriate care.	Otherwise, efforts to change current performance are difficult to justify.
• Good reasons for believing that current performance could be improved.	Concentrates effort on optimum elements of care.

Target criteria and standards

In measuring performance, explicit statements are needed about what to measure (i.e. the audit criteria) and what level of performance is expected (i.e. the standard). Criteria and standards are often confused. Criteria have been defined as 'systematically developed statements that can be used to assess the appropriateness of health care decisions, services and outcomes' (Institute of Medicine, 1992). On the other hand, a standard is: 'The percentage of events that should comply with the criterion' (Baker and Fraser, 1995).

If measurements of actual performance in an audit are to be meaningful and of practical value it is of fundamental importance that the audit criteria against which actual performance is to be judged are developed in compliance with the following four key principles (Baker and Fraser, 1995). Audit criteria must be:

- based on evidence;
- prioritized;
- measurable;
- appropriate to the setting.

Based on evidence

Since audit review criteria are the 'gold standard' against which performance is to be judged, it is of overriding importance, as well as being self-evident, that they must be authoritative. To achieve this status they must be based on the best available current research evidence. Although 'searching the literature' is a skilled and time-consuming activity, it is greatly to be preferred to reliance on unsubstantiated opinions and anecdote. Although few GPs will have the time or inclination to conduct systematic reviews of literature (for example, some 18 000 papers have been published on hypertension since 1989; Fraser *et al.*, 1997), we shall describe in detail in Chapter 2 the methods we employ for identifying evidence-based audit criteria in order to inform readers of the process.

Prioritized according to strength of research evidence and impact on outcome

Some elements of care are supported by more convincing evidence than others. In assessing performance, it would be inappropriate to place the same weight on criteria that are supported only by moderate evidence as those supported by strong evidence. Similarly, various elements of care can have a differential impact on the outcome of care, although they may be supported by equally convincing research evidence. For example, one type of oral contraceptive may carry a higher risk of venous thrombosis than another, but smoking habits are much more important in influencing the likelihood of this outcome. Therefore, a criterion relating to smoking has more impact on outcome, and is therefore more important, than one relating to choice of oral contraceptive. For these reasons, criteria should be prioritized according to the impact on outcome and strength of evidence.

We would suggest that there are three potential categories of priority of audit criteria (Baker and Fraser, 1995). The first we have called 'must do'. Criteria in this category have an important impact on outcome and are supported by convincing research evidence. Criteria classified as 'should do' have less impact on outcome and may also be supported by less strong research evidence. At the margins it involves professional judgement to assign particular criteria to one of these two categories. 'Could do' criteria make up the third category, as they have minimal impact on outcome as well as lacking research evidence. Accordingly, we would recommend that 'could do' criteria should not be routinely included in audits, as appropriate clinical practice is uncertain. This ensures that participants can concentrate their efforts on the most important aspects of care and associated clinical behaviour.

Measurable

Two essential components of audit are a measurement of performance and a comparison of that performance against target criteria. It follows, therefore, that all selected review criteria must be capable of being measured. Furthermore, in order to ensure that multiple participants in an audit *measure the same thing*, the wording of audit criteria must be sufficiently explicit to minimize opportunities for misunderstanding.

For example, the following criterion, as stated, is liable to cause confusion: 'In patients with hypertension the blood pressure must be measured twice a year'. First, hypertension must be clearly defined. Second, 'twice a year' could include two blood pressure measurements taken at intervals of 2 days or 11 months. Third, where the information is to be recorded is not clear. Finally, it is not explicit whether a statement in the patient record noting that the blood pressure had been checked would suffice or whether the blood pressure level itself should be recorded. Preceded by a clear definition of hypertension, a more explicit and measurable criterion would be: 'The records show that in the last 12 months, the blood pressure level has been recorded at least twice at 6-monthly intervals'.

Appropriate to the clinical setting

Clinical performance must be related to clinical probabilities which in turn are related to context. Accordingly, audit criteria must be appropriate to the setting in which they are to be used. For example, patients attending hospital outpatient departments are a highly selected group in comparison with those attending their GPs. Accordingly, patients with hypertension who are referred to hospital are more likely to have secondary causes for their condition and a wide range of investigations may be warranted. However, such investigations, properly indicated in a hospital-referred population, are much less likely to be appropriate for hypertensive patients attending their GP.

Setting standards

In setting standards, it is essential that they are realistic and attainable rather than idealistic and impossible to achieve in the 'real world'. This, however, should not be used as an excuse for setting artificially low standards. For some criteria it may well be reasonable to set the standard at 100 per cent compliance, for example in setting a target of recording at least two blood pressure readings per annum in hypertensive patients. On the other hand, it would be unrealistic to expect all these blood pressure readings to be within ideal limits. Accordingly, it would be more realistic to set the expected standard at less than 100 per cent, the exact figure to depend on local circumstances. Furthermore, it may be appropriate in some instances to set interim standards and gradually increase these on an annual basis until the ultimately desired target is reached.

Data collection

An appropriate and reliable method of collecting data must be devised using a methodology which engenders confidence in their accuracy. The principles of data collection are further discussed in Chapter 3. The 'golden rule', however, is to limit the duration of any data collection to an appropriate minimum, as enthusiasm and efficiency are inversely related to the duration of data collection. This will ensure that data collection does not become so intensive that fatigue overcomes enthusiasm.

Choosing a strategy to implement appropriate change

Many strategies can be used to change performance. Feedback of findings from the first data collection is often the starting point and *can* be highly effective, as it enables the participants to identify deficiencies and make appropriate plans for change in professional behaviour. Nevertheless, feedback alone will not always be sufficient (Grimshaw *et al.*, 1995). A selection of other common practical strategies that can be used is included in Box 1.4. It should be borne in mind, however, that strategies need to be chosen to match the particular circumstances of the audit and its participants.

Box 1.4 Common strategies for implementing change in primary health	
Strategy	**Examples**
Education/training	• In-practice team seminars. • Sessions for individual team members outside the practice. • Visits to the practice by educators, e.g. specialist nurses, consultants. • Sabbaticals for team members.
System changes	• Revised appointment system. • New asthma clinic run by a trained nurse. • Additional telephone line.
Reminder systems	• Posters for team members in the treatment room, e.g. travel immunization. • Structured data entry in computerized records. • Structured paper records, e.g. stamps, special record cards.
Policies/guidelines	• New policy for urgent appointments, agreed at a meeting. • Adoption of new national guideline on management of patients with asthma.
Team changes	• Arrangement for an external facilitator to help the team improve communication and decision making. • Appointment of new staff. • Creation of multidisciplinary sub-groups to develop aspects of care, e.g. a diabetes group, an obstetric group.

Completing the audit cycle

After an appropriate interval, a further period of data collection is required to determine the extent to which the changes which have been implemented have resulted in improvements in standards of care delivered. This stage must not be omitted since no change strategy is so effective that it can be assumed to have worked. The same data as before must be collected and they must again be objective and accurate. If standards have not been met, it may be appropriate either to review them and/or adopt alternative strategies to implement the required changes. Even when satisfactory change has been demonstrated there is a tendency for subsequent performance to decline over time (Fraser *et al.*, 1996). It is for this reason that some people prefer the term audit spiral to audit cycle, as it may be necessary to 'revisit' particular audit topics on future occasions in order to maintain improvements.

Does audit work?

'The audit cycle has become a vicious circle, a noose to strangle any chance of it ever being a practical everyday tool.'

(Farrell, 1995)

'Against a background of rapid change, and in some cases considerable disruption, clinical audit has become a part of everyday life for most health care professionals.'

(Teasdale, 1996)

These two statements were published in the same medical journal within a short time of each other. How can they be reconciled?

Since audit has been adopted, on a voluntary basis, by the great majority of GPs, they must regard it as being of value. What objective evidence is there that participation in systematic audit is an effective way of improving patient care?

Firstly, it is essential to distinguish between the audit cycle as a method and the way it has (frequently) been (mis)applied. Properly applied, using research-based criteria and a systematic approach, there is growing evidence of the potential and actual effectiveness of audit, allied to a variety of implementation strategies, as a means of improving standards of care. The evidence is based on randomized controlled trials (RCTs), systematic reviews of the literature and reports from practices and MAAGs of particular audit projects.

By these means, it has been demonstrated that audit plus feedback of results as a method of implementing change can be enhanced by linking this approach to the use of protocols and educational interventions (Grimshaw *et al.*, 1995; Davis *et al.*, 1995). In a RCT involving groups of trainers, changes in the management of five common childhood conditions brought about improvements, although standard setting was found to be more effective than feedback alone (North of England Study, 1992). In a trial of the audit of digoxin use in five general practices, improvements took place in the care provided by the doctors who took part in the organization of the audit but not their partners (Anderson *et al.*, 1988). Furthermore, in a trial of educational meetings combined with feedback, improvements did take place (Harris *et al.*, 1984) but were not sustained once the interventions were withdrawn (Harris *et al.*, 1985).

The use of practice-based educational meetings to implement guidelines has been shown to be effective (Feder *et al.*, 1995), as was an audit facilitator in assisting practices to improve the monitoring of children with asthma (Bryce *et al.*, 1995). Paper reminders in general practice records have also been shown, albeit in a limited way, to enhance the impact of feedback in an audit of the management of patients taking benzodiazepines (Baker *et al.*, 1997).

Further evidence of the positive impact of audit comes from the many reports of multipractice audits conducted by MAAGs (Baker *et al.*, 1995). In these, MAAGs select a topic, devise an audit protocol, provide practices with instructions for data collection, undertake analysis of the data and return anonymized feedback to practices. This enables practices to compare their performance with that of local colleagues, and encourages appropriate changes in professional behaviour and completion of the cycle of audit. The two commonest topics for multi-practice audits relate to the care of patients with diabetes and asthma respectively. Between 1991 and 1994, 68 MAAGs involved 1700 practices in diabetes audits; the corresponding figures for asthma audits were 53 MAAGs and 1320 practices (Baker *et al.*, 1995). Collated results confirm improvements in both management and outcome of care for both topics. Improvements in care have also been reported with other topics. For example, in an audit of benzodiazepine use involving 3234 patients from 15 practices, drug dependence was reduced by 16 per cent (Holden *et al.*, 1994); another audit involving 1714 patients from 75 practices achieved an approximate reduction of 32 per cent in the frequency of vitamin B12 injections (Fraser *et al.*, 1995).

Thus, the available – and growing – evidence suggests that participation in audit, allied to appropriate implementation strategies, does have a considerable potential for promoting changes in professional behaviour leading to improved outcomes for patients – at least in the short term. Allied to the widely recognized educational potential of audit (Coles, 1989), it is reasonable to conclude therefore that audit does work.

Evidence-based medicine and clinical audit

One of the major trends in current medical practice is the move towards evidence-based medicine. Evidence-based medicine has been defined as 'the conscientious, explicit and judicious use of current best evidence in making decisions about the care of individual patients' (Sackett *et al.*, 1997). In plain language, this means that clinicians are called upon to base their personal practice, wherever possible, on objective research evidence of best practice, even when this conflicts with their past or current professional habits. There is a clear link, moreover, between the practice of evidence-based medicine and participation in clinical audit. Indeed, involvement in audit is acknowledged by the proponents of evidence-based medicine as an essential activity.

The central feature of audit is the gathering of objective evidence of performance which can then be compared with explicit criteria of good practice. This removes the need to rely on unsubstantiated opinions and impressions because it exposes the gap between what we *think* we know and are doing and what we *actually* know and are doing. Accordingly, the audit criteria against which performance is to be reviewed must also be evidence-based. Thus, participation in clinical audit is not only an integral part of evidence-based practice, it also provides the essential framework within which feedback and other implementation strategies for evidence-based practice must be used.

The key activity in identifying and collating up-to-date research evidence on which to base evidence-based practice or audit is the systematic review of the available literature. This is a time-consuming and complex process, and it is sufficient for the purposes of this book to provide a brief outline of the essential steps in conducting a systematic review (Chalmers and Altman, 1995; and see Box 1.5).

Box 1.5 Steps in undertaking a systematic review

- Aims clearly formulated.
- Comprehensive search for studies undertaken using explicit and transparent search strategies.
- Critical appraisal of studies identified.
- Studies selectively included depending on their relevance and quality.
- Data extracted from the studies.
- When possible, the data from similar studies are synthesized statistically (meta-analysis).
- Interpretation of results and conclusions.

One of the reasons why health professionals often fail to apply the findings of research evidence in routine practice has been the failure of traditional reviews and textbooks to take note of up-to-date evidence. This problem has been illustrated by the 10 year delay in the widespread adoption of thrombolysis treatment in acute myocardial infarction. Had a systematic review been undertaken, it would have shown decisive evidence of the value of the treatment at an earlier stage (Antman *et al.*, 1992). Consequently, audits of the care of patients who have suffered a myocardial infarction undertaken *after* the publication of the original research but *before* the effectiveness of thrombolysis was widely recognized would have failed to encourage desired clinical behaviour and optimal patient outcomes. This illustrates and reinforces the need to incorporate up-to-date evidence in audit protocols.

Key points

- Audit is the process of critically and systematically assessing our own professional activities with a commitment to improving personal performance and ultimately the quality and/or cost-effectiveness of patient care.

- Systematic audit has a number of essential stages which should be carried out sequentially: topic selection; identification of specific aims; specification of desired performance in terms of criteria and standards; collection of data to facilitate comparison of actual and desired performance; selection of an appropriate strategy to implement required change in performance; further data collection to evaluate the extent of change.

- There is convincing evidence that systematic audit can lead to change, particularly when linked to explicit criteria and standards and appropriate implementation strategies.

- Criteria against which performance is to be judged should be based on research evidence, prioritized according to the strength of the evidence and impact on outcome, be measurable and appropriate to the clinical setting.

- Participation in audit is probably the most effective way of enabling GPs and primary health care teams to monitor and improve the quality of care they deliver to their patients.

References

Anderson, C.M., Cambers, S., Clamp, M. *et al.* (1988) Can audit improve patient care? Effects of studying use of digoxin in general practice. *BMJ* **297**: 113–114.

Antman, E.M., Lau, J., Kupelnick, B. *et al.* (1992) A comparison of results of meta-analysis of randomised controlled trials and recommendations of experts. *JAMA* **268**: 240–248.

Baker, R. and Fraser, R.C. (1995) Development of review criteria: linking guidelines and assessment of quality. *BMJ* **311**: 370–373.

Baker, R., Hearnshaw, H., Cooper, A. *et al.* (1995) Assessing the work of medical audit advisory groups in promoting audit in general practice. *Quality in Health Care* **4**: 234–239.

Baker, R., Farooqi, A., Tait, C. and Walsh, S. (1997) Randomised controlled trial of reminders to enhance the impact of audit in general practice on management of patients who use benzodiazepines. *Quality in Health Care* **6**: 14–18.

Bryce, F.P., Neville, R.G., Crombie, I.K. *et al.* (1995) Controlled trial of an audit facilitator in diagnosis and treatment of childhood asthma in general practice. *BMJ* **310**: 838–842.

Chalmers, I. and Altman, D.G. (1995) *Systematic Reviews*. London: BMJ Publishing Group.

Coles, C. (1989) Self-assessment and medical audit: an educational approach. *BMJ* **299**: 807–808.

Crombie, I.K., Davies, H.T.O., Abraham, S.C.S. and Florey, C. du V. (1993) *The Audit Handbook*. Chichester: John Wiley and Sons.

Davis, D.A., Thompson, M.A., Oxman, A.D. and Haynes, R.B. (1995) Changing physician performance. A systematic review of the effect of the continuing medical education strategies. *JAMA* **274**: 700–705.

Farrell, L (1995) Audit my shorts. *BMJ* **311**: 1171.

Feder, G., Griffiths, C., Highton, C. *et al.* (1995) Do clinical guidelines introduced with practice based education improve care of asthmatic and diabetic patients? A randomised controlled trial in general practices in east London. *BMJ* **311**: 1473–1478.

Fraser, R.C. (1981) Audit at work – the future. *BMJ* **282**: 1199–1220.

Fraser, R.C. (1982) Medical audit in general practice. *Trainee* **2**: 113–115

Fraser, R.C. Farooqi, A. and Sorrie, R. (1995) Use of vitamin B_{12} in Leicestershire practices: a single topic audit led by a medical audit advisory group. *BMJ* **204**: 1080–1082.

Fraser, R.C., Farooqi, A. and Sorrie, R. (1996) Assessing the long term impact of a complete audit in general practice: a follow-up after 11 years. *Audit Trends* **4**: 125–128.

Fraser, R.C. and Gosling, J.T.L. (1985) Information systems for general practitioners for quality assessment: responses of the doctors. *BMJ* **291**: 1473–1476.

Fraser, R.C., Khunti, K., Baker, R. and Lakhani, M. (1997). Effective audit in general practice: a method for systematically developing audit protocols containing evidence-based review criteria. *Br. J. Gen. Pract.* **47**: 743–746.

Grimshaw, J., Freemantle, N., Wallace, S. *et al.* (1995) Developing and implementing clinical practice guidelines. *Quality in Health Care* **4**: 55–64.

Harris, C.M., Jarman, B., Woodman, E. *et al.* (1984) Prescribing – a suitable case for treatment. Occasional paper 24. London: Royal College of General Practitioners.

Harris, C.M., Fry, J., Jarman, B. and Woodman, E. (1985) Prescribing – a case for prolonged treatment. *J. Roy. Coll. Gen. Pract.* **35**: 284–287.

Holden, J., Hughes, I.M. and Tree, A. (1994) Benzodiazepine prescribing and withdrawal for 3234 patients in 15 general practices. *Family Practice* **11**: 358–362.

Humphrey, C. and Berrow, D. (1993) Developing role of medical audit advisory groups. *Quality in Health Care* **2**: 232–238.

Institute of Medicine (1992) *Guidelines for Clinical Practice. From Development to Use* (Eds Field, M. and Lohr, K.N.) Washington, DC: National Academy Press.

Irvine, D.H. (1983) Quality of care in general practice: our outstanding problem. *J. Roy. Coll. Gen. Pract.* **33**: 521–523.

Marinker, M. (1990). Principles. In *Medical Audit and General Practice* (Ed. Marinker, M), pp. 1–14. London: BMJ Publishing Group.

NHS Executive (1996a) Clinical Audit in the NHS. Leeds: NHS Executive.

NHS Executive (1996b) Promoting Clinical Effectiveness. A framework for action in and through the NHS. Leeds: NHS Executive.

North of England Study of Standards and Performance in General Practice (1992) Medical audit in general practice: effects on doctors' clinical behaviour and the health of patients with common childhood conditions. *BMJ* **304**: 1480–1488.

Primary Health Care Clinical Audit Working Group of Clinical Outcomes Group (1995) Clinical audit in primary health care: Report to Clinical Outcomes Group. Leeds: NHS Executive

Royal College of General Practitioners (1977) Evidence to the Royal Commission on the National Health Service. *J. Roy. Coll. Gen. Pract.* **27**: 197–206.

Royal Commission on the National Health Service (1979) Report of the Royal Commission on the NHS. HMSO: London.

Sackett, D.G., Richardson, W.S., Rosenburg, W. and Haynes, R.B. (1997) *Evidence-based Medicine. How to Practice and Teach Evidence-based Medicine*. London: Churchill Livingstone.

Secretaries of State for Health, England, Wales, Northern Ireland and Scotland (1989) *Working for Patients*. London: HMSO.

Teasdale, S. (1996) The future of clinical audit: learning to work together. *BMJ* **313**: 574.

Developing evidence-based audit criteria and protocols

Introduction

In Chapter 1 we highlighted the four key principles to be followed in deriving audit criteria against which actual performance is to be judged: audit criteria should be evidence-based, prioritized, measurable and appropriate to the clinical setting. In this chapter, we will describe how audit criteria, based on these principles, can be derived and incorporated into protocols which also include instructions and documentation to assist audit participants to complete the cycle of audit in a systematic way. By providing an insight into audit protocol construction, it is our hope that readers will be more prepared to use such protocols – if available and suitable – in preference to spending valuable time trying to construct their own. As we shall see, constructing audit protocols is a highly skilled and time-consuming activity which few practitioners are likely to have the time or inclination to undertake. Furthermore, there is convincing evidence that most GPs and MAAGs are perfectly happy to use externally developed audit protocols constructed according to the principles outlined above (Baker and Fraser, 1997).

Audit criteria are the core feature of any systematic approach to audit. One of the first recorded uses of audit criteria was by a public health physician in the USA in an audit of major female pelvic surgery (Lembcke, 1956). The criteria were identified from respected textbooks of the period, an approach that would be criticized today; nevertheless, there was a reduction in the proportion of inappropriate operations in the participating hospital which was not replicated in non-participating hospitals.

Ten years later Donabedian (1966) produced a useful conceptual framework for assessing quality of care in terms of three categories of criteria: structure, process and outcome. Criteria of structure refer to the resources of a health care system such as equipment, personnel and facilities. Process criteria relate to the activities undertaken by health care staff, such as consultations, technical procedures, referral of patients and the prescription of medication. Outcome criteria refer to changes in the health status of patients due to antecedent care, for example, improvement in symptoms, levels of complications, life expectancy etc.

Although measurement of structural criteria is the easiest to achieve, in the context of clinical audit it is a poor predictor of the quality of clinical care. Conversely, outcome criteria are usually the most difficult to determine, but when this is possible they can be sensitive indicators of quality. Nevertheless, both process and outcome criteria can provide valid and useful information about the quality of care delivered.

It needs to be remembered, however, that many other factors influence the outcome of clinical care in addition to the care provided by health professionals (Brook *et al.*, 1996). Thus, a poor outcome is not necessarily the result of poor care; for example, a diabetic patient may have received exemplary care but may still develop complications. Therefore, process criteria are the most sensitive reflectors of professional performance. Accordingly, it is perfectly appropriate that they are the most commonly selected audit criteria particularly if it can be shown that they are important determinants of outcome. For example, it is well established that if patients are fully immunized against tetanus it is impossible for them to contract the disease. In such circumstances it is necessary only to measure the *process* of immunization of patients against tetanus to be able to predict a satisfactory *outcome* with confidence. In this case the relationship between process and outcome is so well established that process criteria of this type can be regarded as 'intermediate outcomes'. In order to reflect and measure professional performance in general practice we would, therefore, agree that most audits should concentrate on evaluating the process of care (Brook *et al.*, 1996).

Box 2.1   Types of criteria

- Implicit   A health professional's personal, unwritten criteria, not specified before the audit.
- Explicit   Specified in writing in advance of the audit.

Criteria may be implicit or explicit (see Box. 2.1). Implicit criteria have major weaknesses, however, which makes them unsuitable for use in clinical audit. They not only place too much weight on the (potentially idiosyncratic) opinions of the assessor(s) but they may also not be applied consistently by individual or multiple assessors. Consequently, audit participants using implicit criteria have no guarantee that the results of the audit are valid, i.e. that they represent the true state of affairs.

As this greatly diminishes the demonstrable impact of the audit, we would recommend strongly that explicit criteria should be used if audit participation is to be meaningful. How are explicit audit criteria identified?

The systematic identification of audit criteria

Although the ways in which audit criteria have been identified have undergone substantial changes over the past 40 years, the general trend has been increasingly to adopt a more systematic and evidence-based approach. The earliest approaches were based on the utilization of information from textbooks (often out of date) and largely unstructured inputs from 'experts'. The next stage was the creation of expert panels which used more or less formal procedures for reaching consensus. In the past 10 years such panels have made increasing use of systematic literature reviews to inform their discussions. The most recent development has been to make use of the increasing output of evidence-based clinical guidelines by converting elements of these guidelines into audit criteria and then incorporating them in audit protocols.

Although there are many shared steps in the creation of evidence-based guidelines or audit criteria, it is important to be aware that guidelines and audit criteria are *not* synonymous (see Box 2.2).

Box 2.2 Definitions of guidelines, criteria and protocols for clinical practice	
Clinical guidelines	Systematically developed statements to assist practitioner and patient decisions about appropriate health care for specific clinical circumstances[a].
Audit criteria	Systematically developed statements that can be used to assess the appropriateness of specific health care decisions, services and outcomes[a].
Audit protocol	A comprehensive set of criteria for a single clinical condition or aspect of organization[b].

[a] Institute of Medicine (1992)
[b] Baker and Fraser (1995)

Clinical guidelines are used *prospectively* to aid decision making, whereas audit criteria are used *retrospectively* in the assessment of decision-making and performance that have already taken place. Although related, the respective roles of guidelines and criteria can be clarified by the following example. The guidelines of the British Hypertension Society state: 'Great emphasis should be placed on encouraging patients to stop smoking, as the coexistence of smoking as an additional risk factor in hypertensive patients confers a much increased risk of subsequent cardiovascular events'.

To convert this guideline into audit criteria it would need to become: The records show that at least annually, (a) there has been an assessment of smoking habit and (b) appropriate advice has been given to smokers. The audit criteria thus derived from the original guideline make clear what information is required to assess clinical compliance, how the information is to be obtained and the time period in which smoking habits should be assessed. It illustrates how criteria *used for assessment* need to be more detailed and specific than guidelines' statements *used to assist decision making*.

Nevertheless, it is often difficult to derive audit criteria directly from guidelines for two principal reasons. First, guidelines generally include recommendations about every element of care of the condition concerned, without prioritizing their impact on outcomes. For example, the North of England evidence-based angina guidelines (North of England Evidence-Based Guideline Development Project, 1996) has 60 recommendations, whereas the Lilly Centre angina audit protocol has only seven 'must do' criteria (Khunti *et al.*, 1995). This illustrates that in making judgements about the quality of care, it is fundamental to place greatest weight on those key elements of care which are most influential. Secondly, guideline recommendations are usually based on research evidence *and* (inevitably) the values and opinions of the guideline panel (Hayward *et al.*, 1995). Frequently, however, these values are not made explicit, and without directly consulting primary sources of research evidence it is not usually possible to assess the relative importance of particular recommendations in terms of strength of evidence and impact on outcome.

Although a considerable literature exists on methods for developing and using clinical guidelines (Hadorn and Baker, 1994), ways of developing evidence-based audit criteria have received less attention. As a consequence, we have devised a six-stage method for developing audit criteria and incorporating them in audit protocols (see Box 2.3).

Box 2.3   Six-stage method for developing audit criteria and protocols

- Selection of a topic.
- Identification of the key elements of care.
- Focused systematic literature reviews to develop, when justified by evidence, one or more criteria for each element of care.
- Prioritization of the criteria on the strength of research evidence and impact on outcome.
- Incorporation of the criteria in a protocol.
- Submission of the protocol to external peer review.

This systematic approach facilitates critical appraisal of the available evidence and its conversion into prioritized review criteria. Furthermore, by linking explicit criteria to the evidence by the inclusion of descriptive text in the audit protocol, it makes clear why each criterion has been included, highlights the most important and allows potential users to fully understand the steps taken in their development.

The methods that we use will now be described and exemplified with reference to our protocol for the management of hypertension in primary care (Lakhani *et al.*, 1995). [This section of the chapter is based largely on our recent report outlining the details of the method

(Fraser *et al.*, 1997) and appears by kind permission of the Editor of the *British Journal of General Practice*.]

Selection of a topic

Efforts to improve quality should be concentrated on those topics for which compliance with research evidence would lead to the greatest improvements in health. As a preliminary requirement, therefore, potential topics must first satisfy the four principles outlined in Chapter 1 (see Box 1.2).

Identifying the key elements of care

If a clinical topic is chosen, all the elements of care relevant to its diagnosis and patient management must be identified. For example, in any audit of the care of patients with asthma it must first be established that patients labelled and treated as asthmatics actually have reversible airways obstruction. As a consequence, a fundamental element of care will be an explicit statement of the symptoms and signs that patients need to satisfy to be regarded as truly suffering from asthma. Appropriate elements of care relating to management would include criteria for assessing symptom control, medication, patient compliance, frequency of patient review etc.

To ensure that no element of care is overlooked, use is made, whenever possible, of research-based guidelines and/or good quality systematic reviews such as those produced by the NHS Centre for Reviews and Dissemination or the Cochrane Collaboration. If research evidence is lacking we believe it is preferable not to proceed with the development of audit criteria. The identification of the key elements of care in the Lilly Centre protocol on the management of patients with hypertension (Lakhani *et al.*, 1995), as shown in Box 2.4, was greatly assisted by the availability of some authoritative reviews and guidelines (Sever *et al.*, 1993; WHO/ISH, 1993),

---

Box 2.4 Key elements of care of patients with hypertension
- Definition of hypertension; treatment thresholds.
- Measurement of BP: equipment, technique, ambulatory blood pressure monitoring.
- Clinical evaluation.
- Target organ damage evaluation.
- Assessment of risk factors.
- Investigations in general practice.
- Non-pharmacological treatment.
- Drug treatment.
- Quality of life on drugs.
- Organization of care.
- Follow-up intervals.
- Target blood pressure.

Ownership through local development appears to be less important, therefore, than the credibility and perceived utility of externally produced audit protocols (see Box 2.1). Ownership in audit activities is more likely to be satisfied by participants being the prime movers in selecting the particular audit topic and exercising their right to set local standards to take account of local factors. Accordingly, the time and energies of practitioners and primary health care team members can best be used by availing themselves of appropriately designed audit protocols, whatever their origin, rather than attempting to design their own.

Key points

- The identification of explicit audit criteria is the core feature of any systematic approach to audit.

- Most audits should focus on the process of care since the most practical method of assessing the quality of care delivered by health professionals is to compare their performance against explicit evidence-based process criteria.

- The identification of evidence-based and prioritized audit criteria and their incorporation in audit protocols are time-consuming and skilled activities.

- There are important differences between clinical guidelines and audit criteria.

- The perceived utility and credibility of externally developed audit criteria and protocols are more important than ownership through local production.

- Whenever possible practitioners should concentrate their efforts on using appropriately designed and externally developed audit protocols rather than attempting to produce their own.

References

Alderman, M. (1994) Non-pharmacological treatment of hypertension. *Lancet* **244**: 307–311.

Antman, E.M., Lao, J., Kupelnick, B. *et al.* (1992) A comparison of results of meta-analyses of randomised control trials and recommendations of clinical experts. *JAMA* **268**: 724–728.

Baker, R. and Fraser, R.C. (1995) Development of review criteria: linking guidelines and assessment of quality. *BMJ* **311**: 370–373.

Baker, R. and Fraser, R.C. (1997) Is ownership more important than the scientific credibility of audit protocols? A survey of medical audit advisory groups. *Family Practice* **14**: 107–111.

Brook, R.H., McGlynn, E.A. and Cleary, P.D. (1996) Measuring quality of care. *N. Engl. J. Med.* **335** (13): 966–970.

Cutler, J.A., Follman, D., Elliot, P. *et al.* (1991) An overview of randomised trials of sodium reduction and blood pressure. *Hypertension* **17** (Suppl.): I-27–33.

Donabedian, A. (1966) Evaluating the quality of medical care. *Millbank Memorial Fund Quarterly* **44**: 166–203.

Fraser, R.C., Khunti, K., Baker, R. and Lakhani, M. (1997) Effective audit in general practice: a method for systematically developing audit protocols containing evidence-based review criteria. *Br. J. Gen. Pract.* **47**: 743–746.

Grimshaw, J., Freemantle, N., Wallace, S. *et al.* (1995). Developing and implementing clinical practice guidelines. *Quality in Health Care* **4**: 55–64.

Hadorn, D.C. and Baker, D. (1994) Development of the AHCPR–Sponsored Heart Failure Guideline: Methodology and Procedural Issues. *J. Quality Improvement* **20**: 539–547.

Hayward, R.S.A., Wilson, M.C., Tunis, S.R. *et al.* (for the evidence-based medicine working group (1995) Users' guides to the medical literature. VII. How to use clinical practice guidelines. A. Are the recommendations valid? *JAMA* **274**: 570–574.

Institute of Medicine (1992) *Guidelines for Clinical Practice. From Development to Use* (Eds Field, M.J. and Lohr, K.N.) Washington, DC: National Academy Press.

Isles, C.G., Walker, L.M., Beevers, D.G. *et al.* (1996) Mortality in patients of the Glasgow blood pressure clinic. *J. Hypertension* **4**: 141–156.

Khunti, K., Baker, R. and Lakhani, M. (1995) *Management of Angina in General Practice.* Leicester: Eli Lilly National Clinical Audit Centre, University of Leicester.

Lakhani, M., Baker, R. and Khunti, K. (1995) *Management of Hypertension in Primary Care.* Leicester: Eli Lilly National Clinical Audit Centre, University of Leicester.

Law, M.R., Frost, C.D. and Wald, N.J. (1991) By how much does dietary salt reduction lower blood pressure? *BMJ* **302**: 819–824.

Lembcke, P.A. (1956) Medical auditing by scientific methods, illustrated by major female pelvic surgery. *JAMA* **162**: 646–655.

North of England Evidence-Based Guideline Development Project (1996) The primary care management of stable angina. Report no. 74. Newcastle: Centre for Health Services Research, University of Newcastle.

Sackett, D.L. (1986) Rules of evidence and clinical recommendations on the use of antithrombotic agents. *Chest* **89**: 2s–3s.

Sackett, D.L., Haynes, R.B. and Tugwell, P. (1991) *Clinical Epidemiology*, 2nd Edn. Boston, MA: Little Brown and Co.

Sever, P., Beevers, G., Bulpitt, C. *et al.* (1993) Management guidelines in essential hypertension: Report on the Second Working Party of the British Hypertension Society. *BMJ* **306**: 983–987.

WHO/ISH Mild Hypertension Liaison Committee (1993) Summary of the World Heart Organisation: International Society of Hypertension guidelines for the management of mild hypertension. *BMJ* **307**: 1541–1546.

Woolf, S.M., Battista, R.N., Aderson, M. *et al.* and The Canadian Task Force on the Periodical Health Examination (1990). Assessing the clinical effectiveness of preventative measures: analytic principles and systematic methods in reviewing evidence and developing clinical practice recommendations. *J. Clin Epidemiol.* **43**: 891–895.

How to carry out an audit in practice

In this chapter we intend to develop some of the themes outlined in Chapter 1 and advise on how to overcome some of the practical difficulties that may be encountered when conducting an audit in real life general practice. The chapter will follow the various stages of the audit cycle, describe the techniques of audit and include some practical examples. The themes covered will include encouraging the team to participate in audit, topic selection, identifying specific aims, agreeing criteria and standards, data collection/analysis, completing the audit cycle by agreeing and implementing changes and repeating the data collection. We will also identify practical sources of advice to assist in the planning and implementing of audit projects.

Key steps to consider — Encouraging participation

A key step in initiating audit is persuading the practice team to take part, since it is known that audit can evoke a negative or even hostile response from some team members. Consequently, any perceived or actual barriers to audit need first to be identified and then overcome.

Box 3.1 outlines the main barriers to participation and indicates how they can be overcome. When planning an audit, the participants must assign principal responsibility for its organization to an individual participant. This leadership role is essential to maintain enthusiasm and to ensure not only that appropriate steps are taken to overcome any barriers but that each stage is also fully completed (see also Appendix 2).

Box 3.1 Participation – overcoming the barriers

Barrier/problem to participation in audit	Possible solutions
Lack of time	• Audit can save time by addressing issues which cost the practice time, e.g. an audit to reduce unnecessary home visits. • Audit can generate extra income, which may mean extra resources to 'buy' time, e.g. an audit to ensure higher immunization targets are met. • Audit activity can be substituted for less productive time, e.g. earning PGEA credits for in-house audit rather than attending lectures. • The practice may be able to obtain extra resources to help with the audit, e.g. from the local PCAG, Community Trust or directly from the Health Authority. • Task delegation to team members with appropriate skills.
Lack of skills/protocols	• The protocol required may already be available, e.g. from the PCAG, Lilly Audit Centre, Royal Colleges etc. • The local PCAG may help with audit design, data/analysis/interpretation. • Consider training to develop more in-house audit skills, e.g. approach PCAGs for training, attend formal courses.
Negative attitude to audit and general lack of support from practice team.	• Ensure team members understand the definition and purpose of audit. • Enlist the PCAG to help demonstrate the value of audit. • Demonstrate the benefit to colleagues by carrying out a pilot or small-scale audit. • Consider training in team building.

Topic selection

Selecting an appropriate and meaningful topic can be done using a variety of sources, for example suggestions from practice team members, information from practice quality systems (e.g. the patients' complaints procedure), national or health authority defined priorities or new research evidence. Potential topics for audit should first be assessed for their suitability, relevance, priority, practicality and impact. An example of an evaluation form which may help this process is given in Box 3.2 (see also Box 1.2). If the total score is 6 or less it is probably better not to proceed with the proposed audit topic.

Box 3.2   Choosing an audit topic[a]

Questions for scoring topics:

1. Does this address a real problem which is relevant to patient care?
2. Is this problem a priority?
3. Are the data readily accessible and easy to collect?
4. Can the data be collected within a reasonable length of time?
5. If agreed standards are not reached, will you be prepared to implement changes to remedy the problem?

Score: 2 = yes; 1 = not sure; 0 = no.

Topic/ problem	1. A real problem	2. A prio- rity	3. Data to hand	4. Data collection feasible	5. Prepared to change	Total score

[a]Darling and Sorrie, 1993

Defining aims

Clear aims must be identified at the outset of any audit project in order to define its purpose explicitly. This, in turn, helps participants to select the most appropriate methods. Furthermore, it is essential that all involved are familiar with the agreed aim(s) of any particular audit as this improves motivation and compliance. It needs to be remembered that, ultimately, the measure of the success of any particular audit is the extent to which it achieves its defined aims.

Agreeing criteria and target standards

The next stage is to agree the criteria against which the quality of performance is to be judged. This can often generate a considerable debate amongst those involved in the audit. Our advice is to try to utilize already available audit protocols based on prioritized and up-to-date research evidence. If none is available we would advise that you contact your local PCAG for help before attempting to devise your own as this is likely to save you considerable time and effort.

As a practical example, one practice decided to conduct an audit of the care it offered to its diabetic patients. The practice discovered that an evidence-based prioritized audit protocol was already available (see Baker *et al.*, 1993 and Chapter 4). Box 3.3 outlines the 'must do' criteria from that protocol, which the practice was happy to accept. Practices may, of course, modify an externally developed protocol to suit their particular circumstances, but in general must always include all the 'must do' criteria. They may, however, set standards appropriate to their particular context.

Box 3.3 'Must do' criteria for an audit of diabetic care

1. Patients diagnosed as diabetic have been recorded in the practice diabetic register.
2. The records show that diagnosis of diabetes is correct (i.e. a patient labelled as being diabetic must have been shown to have diabetes).

In the last year:

3. The glycated haemoglobin has been checked and the result is within the normal range.
4. The feet have been examined.
5. The patient's urine has been checked for albumin/microalbumin to detect early evidence of nephropathy.
6. The fundi have been examined for retinopathy through dilated pupils.
7. There has been an assessment of smoking habits.
8. The blood pressure has been checked and is within normal limits.

Having selected the necessary criteria, target standards must now be set in order to indicate the level of performance the practice team feels it ought to be achieving for each criterion. The target standard is usually expressed as a percentage, for example: 100 per cent of the practice's diabetic patients will have had their fundi examined in the past 12 months.

According to Crombie *et al.* (1993), standards fulfil three main roles. Firstly, they promote education because health professionals are encouraged to improve their knowledge of the topic being audited. Secondly, the process of comparing current performance with target standards highlights problem areas that may otherwise have gone unheeded. Thirdly, standards are useful as change motivators, especially when the actual performance is found to be lower than the target standards (as is often the case).

A number of factors must be considered when setting standards. First of all participants need to consider the extent to which criteria relate to the process of care (over which they have control) or the outcome of care (over which they may have limited control). For example, although it is desirable that all diabetics should have their smoking status checked it would be unreasonable to expect all to stop smoking, even though the practice personnel delivered exemplary clinical advice and support in an attempt to persuade the patient to stop smoking. 'Must do' criteria carry an implied standard of 100 per cent, but it may not always be possible to achieve perfection. For example, a patient may consistently default from attending the diabetic clinic or optician for retinal examination despite repeated reminders. Secondly, those involved in the audit need to think carefully about what can be practically achieved 'in the real world' where optimum circumstances rarely apply. Consequently, a practice may, quite reasonably, decide to set varying standards for different criteria. As audit is chiefly concerned with continuous quality improvement, the practice may decide to set increasing levels of standard to be achieved over time (so-called stretch standards). Practices should not fall into the trap, however, of setting minimum standards which they know they can readily achieve with little or no effort.

Audit methods

The key to completing a successful audit lies in its planning. It is during this phase that the chosen methodology of the audit must be expressed clearly so that everyone involved understands what is happening and why. The commonest audit methodologies are:

- prospective – collect data as care is given;
- retrospective – collect data after care has been given;
- significant event/critical incident.

Prospective method
A prospective audit should be undertaken if there are no reliable records already available from which to extract the required data; for example, in undertaking an audit of waiting times in surgery. It is likely that a practice will have to design a special data collection form as such information will probably not be routinely collected. The main advantages of using this method are that it ensures economy of effort as data recording is selective and that it is more likely to lead to an accurate picture of the topic or problem being audited. One possible disadvantage is that participants may prematurely alter their behaviour in order to project what they hope will be a more favourable impression. Audit participants need to be warned to guard against this and encouraged to continue 'normal practice' until the first data collection phase is completed. Another disadvantage of prospective data collection is that it relies on members of the team identifying patients. The inevitable pressure of time, or reluctance to include in the audit patients whose care may have been deficient, can result in the identification of fewer patients than expected.

Retrospective method
Retrospective audit involves use of existing data, most commonly held in the medical record, to obtain the necessary information. Theoretically, these data already provide a record of the care or service that was actually provided. However, it is essential to bear in mind that retrospective audits rely both on the completeness and

accuracy of the records from which the data are collected. If this method is to be used, practices must be confident that their routine recording is of an appropriate level of reliability whether held on paper or computer records, otherwise, the audit will not be a true test of level of care delivered.

Significant event/critical incident method
Although this is a variant of true systematic audit, significant event audit shares some of its features such as choosing a topic and identifying change. This approach involves the detailed examination of a single critical episode in the care of a patient, and may encompass both clinical and organizational aspects. The rationale is that problems in the process of care will be revealed and consequently avoided when dealing with future patients who require similar care. Significant events are chosen on the basis that they are considered important and can provide insight into the overall care offered by the practice (Pringle and Bradley, 1994). Examples of significant events are misfiled test results, sudden deaths, urgent visits and correspondence that has not been acted upon. The advantage of significant event auditing is that the information it provides is more qualitative than quantitative and, hence, it does not involve designing data collection forms, and the amassing of large and possibly complicated data sets, nor does it require prolonged analyses. However, in order to be successful, it should not seek to allocate blame to any individual in the practice. It should be regarded more as a learning opportunity. For such a method to be used successfully, all involved members of the team should give their prior agreement to the audit being undertaken and its results should be kept confidential within that team. The disadvantage of the significant event method is that it may not have direct impact on the care of groups of patients. However, the findings may be used as the trigger for a formal systematic audit involving all relevant patients.

Data collection

Before data can be collected systematically and economically, a number of questions must be addressed so that the appropriate method can be identified. These are outlined below.

1. What is the aim of the audit?
This has already been dealt with in Chapter 1; nevertheless, it should again be emphasized that data collection should be restricted to a minimum sufficient to satisfy the aims of the audit.

2. How are the data to be located?
An audit topic can often be defined in terms of a specific patient population, for example all the diabetics on the practice list. In order to identify a target population it may be possible to turn to a number of existing sources within the practice, for example disease registers and repeat prescribing systems, from which some of the

relevant data may be readily collected. For example, the practice may be able to rapidly identify the majority of its diabetic patients because it has an up-to-date diabetic register. Alternatively, a search could be undertaken of the repeat prescribing system to identify patients receiving prescriptions relevant to diabetes, such as urine testing sticks, oral therapies and insulin preparations. Data may also have to be collected opportunistically during the consultation or at the reception desk. Sometimes, external sources can be usefully employed.

3. How many patients should be included in the audit?

In order to conserve the energies and resources of the practice the number of patients to be included in any audit should be the minimum that will provide appropriate results to satisfy the aims. Including all potential patients in the target population, for example the practice's diabetic patients, will obviously provide the most accurate results. This may be appropriate if the total number is small or the data required for the audit are easy to collect. In many instances, however, it is not necessary to scrutinize the entire target population, as sampling can be used. This has the added benefit of reducing the work-load of the audit.

Optimal sample sizes can be calculated using statistical formulae (Samuel *et al.*, 1993) or by consulting a sample size table (Derry, 1993). The following example uses the method recommended by Samuel *et al.* (1993).

Consider again our hypothetical practice which is undertaking an audit of diabetes. They have identified 300 diabetic patients, and feel that collecting data about all these would be a major task: they decide to sample and to base their calculation of sample size on the criterion relating to glycated haemoglobin checks (see Box 3.3), and aim to achieve a standard of 90 per cent. They are willing to accept, within limits, some error as a result of using the sample. They opt for a 10 per cent limit; in other words, if they achieve a standard of 90 per cent in their sample, the true figure is likely to lie between 80 per cent and 100 per cent. Applying these figures to the formula provided by Samuel *et al.* (1993):

$$N = \frac{90(100-90)}{2.5^2}$$

gives a sample size of 144 (where 2.5^2 is the standard error squared, calculated as one quarter of the confidence interval of 10 per cent). Thus, the practice is able to reduce the burden of data collection by one half without sacrificing accuracy.

Nevertheless, it is essential that the sample of patients selected should be typical of the population from which it is drawn. That is, it should be representative of the characteristics and features of the target population, which means that the sample audit results can then be generalized to the whole population.

A wide variety of sampling methods exist, but for the purpose of audit, the following two techniques are the most widely applied:

- 'random' sampling;
- 'systematic' (or quasi-random) sampling.

Whenever possible, we would advise that random sampling should be employed as this is simple to do and is more likely to produce a representative sample.

Random sampling. This method ensures that every patient belonging to the target population of the audit has an equal chance of being included in the sample. It can be illustrated by continuing our example of diabetes audit. All 300 diabetic patients are allocated a number, starting at 1. Random numbers are then used to select the required 144 patients. These numbers can be generated using a computer or by using a random numbers table, which can be found in most statistics textbooks. This consists of columns and rows of randomly listed three digit numbers, for example:

```
 34  162  277
977  844  217
167  630  163
125  332  112
555  576   86 etc.
```

Starting at an arbitrary point in the table, one progresses down the columns and continues to the next group of columns, selecting as many numbers as are required for the sample size. Every time a number between 1 and 300 is found, the patient with the corresponding number is selected. Thus, patients 34, 167, 125, 162, 277, 217, 163, 112 and 86 would be included in the diabetic audit, and so on, until all 144 patients are identified.

Systematic (or quasi-random) sampling. This entails the selection of every nth patient from a finite population. For example, in the audit of diabetic care the practice register of diabetic patients totals 300. It has been estimated that a sample size of 144 patients is appropriate: the first patient should be selected at random and then every second patient should be selected from the diabetic register. This method should generate a reasonably representative sample.

4. How will the data be collected?
Data collection is usually facilitated by designing a data recording form which should be self-explanatory and easy to complete. Only the specific data required for the audit should be collected and all participants should use the same forms. Each form should be dated, so that data can be related to a specific time, and titled to assist in recognition. It is usually helpful to undertake an initial pilot trial of the form in order to ensure that it can capture the required data in a convenient way. Furthermore, it also helps to familiarize participants with what is required of them. All those involved in data collection must also be provided with clear instructions about how to collect the data. It is also worthwhile undertaking checks to ensure that the

forms are being completed correctly and, if required, appropriate feedback can then be provided to the staff responsible for the data collection in order to correct deficiencies. Box 3.4 summarizes some of the key features of data collection form design.

Box 3.4   Designing a data collection form – checklist

A data collection form for audit should:

- Be clear and simple to complete.
- Collect only what is needed for the audit.
- Have a meaningful title.
- Include dates.
- Be piloted.

If the audit is to be realistic and achievable, it is essential to consider the resources available to the practice in terms of staff, facilities and time. Particular tasks should be delegated to the most appropriate staff members. Whenever possible, data collection should be done by administrative staff so that doctors and other health professionals can concentrate on clinical care. It also has to be decided whether data collection will be done manually or using a computer. The duration of data recording also needs to be decided: this should be the minimum time required to collect essential information to minimize the risk of diminishing enthusiasm.

The timing of the audit should be planned to avoid major holiday periods or staff absences. Some practices may find an 'audit recording sheet' to be useful whilst planning the audit (see Box 3.5). This will enable the team to document clearly what is to be done during the audit and who has responsibility for particular tasks.

Data analysis

Once the data collection phase is complete, protected time should be set aside for data analysis, summarizing and presentation of feedback to the team. The aim of analysing the data is to produce evidence which will inform the decisions that need to be made regarding the next stage of the audit cycle – implementing change. Extensive statistical analysis is not usually required; indeed, it is usually sufficient to summarize data by performing simple arithmetical calculations. Data will most commonly be in the form of the proportion of patients whose care complies with the criterion, with possible data items being either 'yes' (criterion complied with), 'no' (criterion not complied with) or 'not known' (data missing). The analysis will show the percentage of 'yes' responses. Only occasionally will other simple analyses be needed, such as:

- **Averages/means** – these are obtained by adding up all the values in a group and then dividing the total by the number of values.

Box 3.5 An example of an audit record sheet for use in practice[a]
Audit Record Sheet

Audit start date:	Audit finish date:
First data collection period:	First data collection period:
Second data collection period:	Second data collection period:
Title of audit:	
Aim of audit:	

Criteria and standards:

Criterion: Standard:

1.

2.

3.

etc.

Identification of data to be collected:

Location: Data items:

(where data are held, e.g. appointments   (required for data collection, e.g.
book, patients notes, etc.)   GP data, patients identified etc.)

---

[a]Darling and Sorrie, 1993

- **Mode** – this is the most frequently occurring value in the set of numbers.
- **Median** – the middle value of a set of numbers. This is calculated by arranging values in order of lowest to highest and then choosing the middle one if the set is odd-numbered or the average of the two middle values if the set is even-numbered.

It is usually only advantageous to calculate modes or medians if there is an extended range of values which includes only a small number of 'outliers'.

Confidence intervals
When undertaking an audit based on a sample of patients it is important to take into account the error in the results that may have occurred. For example, if the observed standard obtained for the criterion concerning annual fundi check was found to be 85 per cent for the sample of 144 diabetic patients, to what extent would this result truly represent the level of fundi checks within the target population as a whole? Confidence intervals can be calculated to

show the probable interval within which the results for the target population will be located. Furthermore, the width of the interval will also indicate the level of precision of the results.

Confidence intervals (C.I.s) can be calculated for samples greater than 5 per cent of the population using the following formula (Jarvis, 1997):

$$\text{C.I.} = P \pm 1.96\sqrt{P\frac{(1-P)}{n} \times \left(\frac{N-n}{N}\right)}$$

Where P = observed sample results (expressed as a proportion) based on a sample size n, and N = the target population size.

The following calculations continue our example of the diabetes audit. Taking the standard achieved for the fundi check (85 per cent) and the sample size of 144 patients, the formula would be:

$$\text{C.I.} = 0.85 \pm 1.96\sqrt{\frac{(0.85)\,(1-0.85)}{144} \times \left(\frac{300-144}{300}\right)}$$

Therefore, for the fundi check, the following results were obtained:

- Criterion – fundi check undertaken in the last 12 months ($n = 144$).
- Observed result – 85 per cent.
- 95% C.I. – 81–89 per cent (85 ± 4 per cent).
- Target standard – 100 per cent.

The findings show that the practice has fallen short of its target standard. It is a convention to refer to the 95% C.I. Put simply, 95% C.I.s imply that there is a 95 per cent chance that the true standard of performance is within the confidence intervals of the observed value.

Results

Once the results of the first data collection have been calculated they should be compared with the agreed target standards for all the audit criteria previously identified. Consideration needs to be given to the most informative way of presenting such results. Frequently, the simplest and most effective way is to present the results in tables (see Box 3.6). This format immediately makes clear the elements of care which most need to be improved, i.e. urinalysis and examination of the feet, as well as the elements of care for which high standards have been achieved, i.e. register entry and accuracy of diagnosis. Alternatively, results could be presented as, or supplemented by, bar charts and graphs. A decision needs to be taken on whether further analysis should be carried out, for example a comparative analysis of the results for patients cared for in general practice and hospital.

Box 3.6   Table showing an example of actual performance against the target standards set for a diabetes audit (*N* = 150)

Criterion	Actual standard: first data collection		Target standard
	n	%	%
1. Patient on diabetic register	148	99	100
2. Diagnosis correct	145	97	100
3. Blood pressure checked	142	95	100
4. Smoking habit checked	138	93	100
5. Glycated haemoglobin checked	133	89	100
6. Fundi examined	127	85	100
7. Feet examined	111	74	100
8. Urine checked	103	69	100

Implementing change

The practice is then faced with one of the most challenging aspects of audit: how to effectively implement necessary changes to improve performance. Figure 3.1 illustrates the possible pathways the practice needs to follow and the nature of decisions regarding standards with which a practice may be faced. The first step is to hold a meeting of all audit participants at which a presentation of the results is made, since feedback of results can be a powerful influence on change. Those present can discuss the implications, agree the changes in clinical

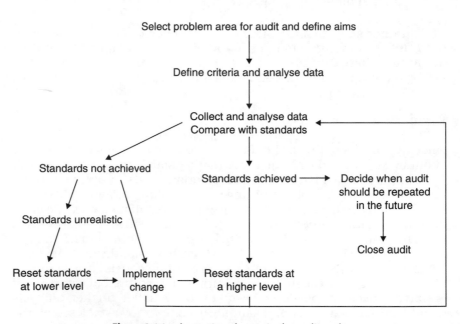

Figure 3.1 Implementing change in the audit cycle

behaviour and/or organization required and identify ways in which such changes should be implemented (see also Box 1.4).

On the other hand, it is likely that the results show that in respect of some of the criteria, the practice has achieved the standards set or is close to doing so. The practice will then need to decide whether it is satisfied with that performance, or if it wishes to achieve a higher standard (if it has initially been set at less than 100 per cent).

If the practice has not achieved one or more of the standards set it will need to consider whether the predefined standards are still reasonable and attainable. If they are, the practice must agree and implement changes to improve performance. Occasionally it may become clear that the standards originally set were too ambitious, in which case new, more realistic, standards should be set.

In the diabetic audit referred to (see Box 3.6) it was decided to concentrate efforts on the following: urinalysis, examination of feet, fundal examination and glycated haemoglobin.

The following practical steps were agreed:

- The introduction of a standard recording form to place in the notes of diabetic patients.
- A seminar for the doctors and practice nurses on diabetes care.
- Use of the register of diabetic patients to co-ordinate annual recall.
- Special training in fundal examinations for one doctor who would in future perform all these examinations on all practice diabetic patients.
- Patients to be routinely asked by the practice nurse to remove their shoes and socks at annual diabetic checks.

The beneficial consequences of such changes can be seen in Box 3.7.

Box 3.7   Results of the practice diabetes audit

Criterion	First data collection (% and 95% C.I.)		Second data collection (% and 95% C.I.)	
1	99	98–100	100	—
2	97	95–99	100	—
3	95	92–98	98	96–100
4	93	90–96	98	96–100
5	89	85–93	96	94–98
6	85	81–89	92	89–95
7	74	69–79	91	88–94
8	69	64–74	87	83–91

Once the cycle has been completed in a particular audit, the practice will have to consider whether and/or when to repeat the process to ensure that standards are maintained. This will depend on a number of issues including importance of the topic, the advent of new evidence which may influence criteria and standards, and the resources and motivation within the practice. In an important condition like diabetes, it would certainly be advisable to have a mechanism in place for re-audit to occur at regular intervals (say every 2 years).

Box 3.8 summarizes the critical points in managing change.

Box 3.8 Managing change – critical points

- Set realistic standards and review these in the light of actual performance as revealed by data collection.
- Managing change will usually be a team process. Therefore, ensure that the change strategy has input and ownership from all involved primary health care team members, e.g. a diabetes audit may involve GPs, receptionists, practice managers, practice nurses and district nurses.
- Audit should not be a 'finger pointing' or blame assigning activity. Use educational principles to demonstrate the need for change.
- Ensure appropriate resource issues are addressed as part of the change management strategy, e.g. administration time to run a call and recall system as part of a diabetes audit.
- Always review your criteria and standards after an appropriate time interval to take account of new evidence.

Support for clinical audit

There are a number of local and national organizations which can support practices wishing to undertake audit. These include Medical Audit Advisory Groups and National Centres.

Medical Audit Advisory Groups (MAAGs)

Since their establishment in 1990, most MAAGs (and equivalent organizations in Scotland and Northern Ireland) have become the key organizations supporting audit in practices. In England and Wales there are some 90 MAAGs, although they now have a variety of titles, including primary care audit groups, multidisciplinary audit groups or clinical effectiveness groups. Their development, remit and resources do vary across the country but most offer a wide range of services to support practices. Their expertise and skills may lie in developing guidelines, undertaking literature surveys, computing (both general systems and dedicated GP computer systems), data handling and statistics. Many have established links with bodies involved in education and research. MAAGs have broadened their focus by becoming involved in issues such as improving practice organization and helping practices to develop their own quality improvement strategies (Berrow et al., 1996). Often this activity seeks to address both professional development and multi-professional working within the primary health care team.

One of the strengths of the MAAG has been its ability to initiate and co-ordinate district wide audits on a single topic. It has been demonstrated that such multipractice audits can encourage large numbers of GPs to take part in audit and can secure meaningful change in clinical practice (Fraser *et al.*, 1995). Most MAAGs which offer this service to general practices will not only analyse and provide feedback of the results to each participating practice on an individual basis, but will also provide anonymized comparative feedback, based on the aggregated data for all participating practices.

National Centres

National Centres, such as the Eli Lilly National Clinical Audit Centre and the National Centre for Clinical Audit, have been established in order to support the development of clinical audit in a variety of ways. This might be through undertaking research on audit and developing evidence-based audit protocols (Lilly Centre) or by establishing a national data base on clinical audit activity (NCCA). Their normal channel of contact with the primary health care team will be through the MAAG or Health Authority.

Key points

- Audit is more likely to be successful if participants have input to all stages of the audit cycle from topic selection through to implementation of change.

- Nevertheless, it is essential to identify one practice member as project leader to maintain enthusiasm and ensure completion of the audit cycle.

- Selected audit topics should be relevant and address areas where improvements are needed.

- Audit criteria, against which actual performance is to be judged, should be evidence-based and prioritized.

- Whenever possible, practices should use readily available audit protocols rather than attempt to devise their own.

- Standards set should be realistic and attainable.

- Data collection should be kept to the minimum necessary to satisfy the aims of the particular audit.

- All participants should be prepared to implement appropriate changes to improve quality standards.

References

Baker, R., Khunti, K. and Lakhani, M. (1993) *Monitoring Diabetes*. Leicester: Eli Lilly National Clinical Audit Centre, University of Leicester.

Berrow, D., Foot, B. and Humphrey, C. (1996) Working together for quality improvement. *Audit Trends* **4**: 53–58

Crombie, I.K., Davies, H.T.O., Abraham, S.C.S. and Florey, C. du V. (1993) *The Audit Handbook*, p. 86. Chichester: John Wiley and Sons.

Darling, L. and Sorrie, R. (1993) *Audit for Teams*. Leicestershire MAAG.

Derry, J. (1993) Sample size for audit. *Managing Audit in General Practice* **1**: 17–20.

Fraser, R.C., Farooqi, A. and Sorrie, R. (1995) Use of vitamin B_{12} in Leicestershire practices: a single topic audit led by a medical audit advisory group. *BMJ* **311**: 28–30

Jarvis, P. (1997) Describing the results of audit, is average enough? *Audit Trends* **5**: 25–27.

Pringle, M. and Bradley, C. (1994) Significant event auditing: a user's guide. *Audit Trends* **2**: 20–23

Samuel, O., Sackin, P. and Sibbald, B. (1993) *Counting on Quality*. London: RCGP.

4

Improving the care of chronic disease: a protocol for an audit of patients with diabetes

Introduction

Diabetes mellitus is one of the commonest chronic conditions encountered in general practice. It has a prevalence of 1–2 per cent (Howitt and Cheales, 1993; Whitford *et al.*, 1995), although it is likely that there is a similar number of undiagnosed diabetics. Diabetes causes substantial morbidity and mortality, has a major impact on lifestyle, and the care of people with diabetes mellitus accounts for 4–5 per cent of the total UK health budget (Leese, 1991).

The Clinical Standards Advisory Group has found unacceptable variations in standards of care and recommended that all people with diabetes should be receiving continuing preventative care from a multidisciplinary diabetes team (Clinical Standards Advisory Group, 1994). Primary care can be as effective as secondary care when judged by commonly used performance measures such as frequency of laboratory tests, frequency of review and measurement of glycated haemoglobin (Greenhalgh, 1994). Although most complications of diabetes are caused by poor blood glucose control in the years following diagnosis, it has been shown that intensive treatment has a beneficial effect on the development and progression of long-term complications in insulin-dependent diabetes (DCCT Research Group, 1993). Box 4.1 summarizes the rationale for auditing diabetes in primary care.

Box 4.1   Rationale for an audit of diabetes

- Diabetes affects large numbers of patients.
- Many patients are cared for entirely in general practice.
- There is evidence of deficiencies in care.
- Better care can improve outcomes for patients.
- There are established clinical guidelines for good care.
- Care of diabetes has substantial cost implications for the practice.

Scope

This protocol has been designed to help practice teams audit the care of patients with both insulin-dependent diabetes (IDDM) and non-insulin-dependent diabetes (NIDDM). The protocol does not include the management of patients with acute illness, nor specific patient groups with particular requirements, for example children, adolescents or pregnant women. However, this protocol will help primary care teams audit the key elements of care of most adult patients with diabetes.

Audit criteria and their justification

The audit criteria have been developed following reference to several guidelines for the management of diabetes, for example from the British Diabetic Association (1993), St Vincent's Task Force (1995) and the Clinical Standards Advisory Group (1994). The key elements of care thus identified included accurate diagnosis and assessment of patient well-being, complications and control. See Box 4.2 for the 'must do' and 'should do' criteria. Only the 'must do' criteria are discussed in detail in this chapter but the evidence relating to 'should do' criteria is available (Baker *et al.*, 1993).

Box 4.2   Audit criteria

'Must do' criteria

- Patients diagnosed as diabetic have been recorded in the practice diabetic register.
- The diagnosis of diabetes is correct (i.e. a patient labelled as being diabetic must have been shown to have diabetes).

The records show that at least annually:

- The glycated haemoglobin has been checked and the result is within the normal range.
- The feet have been examined.
- The patient's urine has been checked for albumin/microalbumin to detect early evidence of nephropathy.
- The fundi have been examined for retinopathy through dilated pupils.
- There has been an assessment of smoking habit.
- The blood pressure has been checked and is within normal limits.

'Should do' criteria

The records show that at least annually:

- There has been an assessment of symptoms including hypoglycaemic attacks and general well-being.
- Each patient will be reviewed at regular intervals agreed with the patient (but not exceeding 12 months).
- Each newly diagnosed patient (or their carer) will receive education about diabetes management.
- The patient's diet has been reviewed.
- The visual acuity has been checked.
- The weight has been checked.
- If the patient normally monitors the condition by urine or blood tests, the technique in performing the tests has been checked.
- The patient's blood or urine monitoring records have been checked.

'Must do' criteria

- *Patients who have been diagnosed as diabetic must be recorded in the practice diabetic register*

A manual or computerized register of affected patients is the cornerstone for systematic care as it enables a practice to identify and systematically plan care for its diabetic patients. Prompting structured care of patients with NIDDM has been shown to be effective and acceptable (Hurwitz *et al.*, 1993).

The register should indicate whether or not patients are receiving insulin and whether they are cared for by the practice alone or by hospital or shared care as this is required for the chronic disease management programme (General Medical Services Committee, 1993). The number of diabetics cared for by an individual GP will vary depending upon the characteristics of the patient list. For example, diabetes is more common in the elderly (Croxon *et al.*, 1991), and the prevalence of diabetes is more common amongst people of Asian or Afro-Caribbean origin (Hawthorne *et al.*, 1993). Accordingly, to check whether your practice has detected a reasonable number of diabetic patients, you must take into account the age distribution and ethnic composition of your practice population.

- *The records show that the diagnosis of diabetes is correct*

It has been demonstrated that nearly 9 per cent of patients being treated as diabetic in one practice did not have diabetes (Patchett and Roberts, 1994). It is essential, therefore, that definitive diagnostic evidence should be sought in the patient record from the time that the patient was first 'labelled' as a diabetic. We would recommend the definitions and diagnostic criteria proposed by the British Diabetic Association (1993) (see Box 4.3).

Box 4.3 Diagnostic criteria for diabetes

	Plasma glucose concentration (mmol/l)		
	Normal	**IGT**[a]	**Diabetes**
Fasting	<7.8	<7.8	≥7.8
OGTT[b]	<7.8	≥7.8–<11.1	>11.1

[a]IGT = impaired glucose tolerance
[b]OGTT = oral glucose tolerance test

- *The records show that the glycated haemoglobin has been checked at least annually and the result is within the normal range*

The glycated haemoglobin value correlates with blood glucose profiles of the previous 4–12 weeks (Paisley *et al.*, 1980), although reference ranges do vary between laboratories (Pickup *et al.*, 1993). Tight control is associated with approximately 60 per cent reduction in the risk of retinopathy, nephropathy and neuropathy in patients with

IDDM (DCCT Research Group, 1993). However, tight control also increases the risk of severe hypoglycaemia and weight gain. The British Diabetic Association offers targets for glycated haemoglobin with the proviso that they may have to be adjusted locally (BDA, 1993) (see Box 4.4).

Box 4.4 Targets for glycated haemoglobin				
	Good	**Acceptable**	**Poor**	**Very poor**
Haemoglobin A_1 normal (5.0–7.5)	<7.5	7.5–8.7	8.8–10	>10
Haemoglobin A_{1c} normal (4.0–6.0)	<6.0	6.0–7.0	7.1–8.1	>8.0

- *The records show that patients who have been diagnosed as having diabetes have had an annual examination of their feet and education about foot care*

Diabetic patients have a 15 times greater risk of lower extremity amputations compared to non-diabetics (Most and Sinnock, 1983), and 30 per cent of patients attending a secondary care diabetic clinic were found to be at risk of diabetic foot complications (Klenerman *et al.*, 1996). Significant correlations with developing a foot complication are: duration of diabetes, age and smoking. NIDDM patients are more at risk of diabetic foot complications than those with IDDM (Klenerman *et al.*, 1996).

Randomised controlled trials (RCTs) in primary care have shown that a structured teaching and treatment programme for NIDDM patients results in a significant reduction in foot lesions and other dermatological abnormalities (Litzelmann *et al.*, 1993). Patients were also more likely to report appropriate foot care behaviours, to have foot examinations during consultations and to receive foot care education from health care providers. The intervention consisted of nurse-clinicians conducting patient education sessions with one to four patients using slide and audio-tape presentations and pamphlets. Another RCT of patients with foot infection, ulceration or prior amputation referred to a podiatry or vascular surgery clinic showed a three-fold reduction in amputation and ulceration rates (Malone *et al.*, 1989).

- *The records show that at least annually the patient's urine has been checked for albumin/microalbumin to detect early evidence of nephropathy*

Unless good care is provided, nephropathy may eventually develop in as many as 35–45 per cent and approximately 20 per cent of patients with IDDM and NIDDM respectively (Ballard *et al.*, 1988). The presence of proteinuria on dip-stick testing heralds the onset of overt or clinical nephropathy.

Most standard dip-sticks give positive results only when the rate of urinary albumin excretion is greater than 360 mg per day (American Diabetes Association, 1994).

Recently, products such as Micral (Boehringer-Mannheim) and the microalbumin test (Ames) have been introduced to detect smaller amounts of albumin; their specificities, however, are fairly low (Tiu *et al.*, 1993). These tests are often used for initial screening, although microalbuminuria is best diagnosed on the basis of quantitative assays (American Diabetes Association, 1994; Tiu *et al.*, 1993). Nevertheless, early detection can make effective treatment of diabetic renal disease possible, or at least progression may be slowed (Mogensen *et al.*, 1995). Studies have demonstrated that screening for microalbuminuria is cost-effective in IDDM (Borch-Johnsen *et al.*, 1993), although no similar analysis has been performed in NIDDM. It is recommended that annual screening for micro-albuminuria is undertaken in patients with IDDM of greater than 5 years' duration (European IDDM Policy Group, 1993) and that all patients with NIDDM have annual screening for albuminuria.

- *The records show that at least annually the fundi have been examined for retinopathy through dilated pupils*

The prevalence of retinopathy reaches more than 90 per cent after 20 years in IDDM (Palmberg *et al.*, 1981) but early treatment can pre-vent blindness in up to 95 per cent of cases of proliferative retino-pathy and 70 per cent of cases of maculopathy (Ferris, 1993). The St Vincent's declaration has therefore set a target of reducing diabetic-related blindness by one third (WHO and International Diabetic Federation, Europe, 1990).

It has been estimated that up to 20 per cent of NIDDM patients already have retinopathy at diagnosis, with 5 per cent needing active treatment (UK Prospective Diabetes Study Group, 1990). Patients with IDDM are at greater risk of retinopathy and visual loss than those with NIDDM (Kohner *et al.*, 1996). In IDDM, careful control can not only reduce the development of retinopathy in patients with no pre-existing retinopathy but can also slow progression in patients with early retinopathy (DCCT Research Group, 1993). In view of this evidence, it has been recommended that screening for retinopathy should take place at annual intervals (Kohner *et al.*, 1996).

- *The records show that at least annually there has been an assessment of smoking habit*

Metabolic control is worse in smokers compared with non-smoking diabetic patients (Dierkx *et al.*, 1996), and smokers with IDDM reported hospitalizations and poor health significantly more fre-quently than non-smokers with or without IDDM (Gay *et al.*, 1992). Furthermore, up to 65 per cent of cardiovascular deaths in smoking diabetic patients could be attributed to the interaction of smoking and diabetes (Dierkx *et al.*, 1996), and smoking is also associated with the development of microvascular complications including nephropathy and retinopathy.

It has been estimated that stopping smoking would be the most effective intervention in reducing the risk of coronary heart disease and would prolong life by a mean of around 3 years in a diabetic man

(Yudkin, 1993). Patients should therefore be advised against smoking and given all necessary assistance in stopping (see Chapter 7).

- *The records show that at least annually the blood pressure has been checked and is within normal limits*

In patients with diabetes, hypertension is defined as blood pressure above 140/90 mmHg (Guidelines Sub-Committee, 1993). The leading causes of morbidity and mortality among patients with hypertension and diabetes are coronary heart disease, stroke, peripheral vascular disease, lower extremity amputations and end-stage renal disease (Fuller *et al.*, 1991a). Hypertension also occurs more frequently in people with diabetes mellitus compared to non-diabetics (Fuller *et al.*, 1991b).

In both IDDM and NIDDM, hypertension has a substantial impact on morbidity and mortality (Yudkin, 1993). Indeed, the relative risks of cardiovascular deaths in NIDDM patients were 2.2 for men and 3.7 for women and in IDDM, 3.5 and 2.5 respectively (Fuller and Head, 1989). Furthermore, it has been estimated that in diabetic men, a 10 year mortality rate from coronary heart disease of 14.4 per 1000 could be reduced to 8.6 per 1000 by antihypertensive treatment (Yudkin, 1993).

Undertaking the audit

Chapter 3 has described in detail how to carry out an audit in practice and included some examples from a diabetes audit. A few additional details are given below.

Identifying patients

You can use your register of diabetic patients if you already have one. If not you must compile a register. Appoint a member of staff to collate a list from the following sources:

- Ask the GPs, practice nurses and other members of the team to identify patients from memory.
- Record the names of diabetics as you encounter them in consultations or on visits. You can issue copies of the patient recording form to doctors and nurses to list patient names.
- Search the repeat prescription system for patients receiving prescriptions for insulin, oral hypoglycaemics, insulin syringes or urine/blood testing reagents.
- You may be able to ask the local diabetic clinic for a list of your patients who attend the hospital.
- Access a district diabetic register if available.

Data collection

Two versions of the data collection form are supplied: one for individual patients and one for 10 patients per form (see Figures 4.1 and

Data collection form   **Diabetes protocol**

Patient code No.	
DOB	
Sex	
Year diagnosed	

Treatment	
Diet only	
Insulin	
NK	
Source of care	
GP only	
Hospital only	
Shared	
NK	

'MUST DO'

Criterion 1

Patient recorded on diabetic register?   y☐   n☐   nk☐

Criterion 2

Diagnosis correct?   y☐   n☐   nk☐

Criterion 3

Glycated Hb checked in past year?   y☐   n☐   nk☐

Result:	normal	☐
	moderately raised	☐
	poor	☐
	nk	☐
If abnormal, action taken:	no action	☐
	change Rx	☐
	refer to hosp	☐
	other	☐

Criterion 4

Feet checked in past year?   y☐   n☐   nk☐

If abnormal, action taken:	advice	☐
	refer to chirop	☐
	refer to hosp	☐
	other	☐

Criterion 5

Urine checked in past year for:

albumin	y☐	n☐	nk☐
microalbumin?	y☐	n☐	nk☐
	result +ve	☐	
	result −ve	☐	
If result +ve:	MSU	☐	
	creatinine	☐	
	other	☐	

Criterion 6

Fundi checked in past year?   y☐ n☐ nk☐

Were the pupils dilated?   y☐   n☐   nk☐

If yes, checked by:	GP	☐
	optician/ optometrist	☐
	hosp diabetic clinic	☐
	hosp ophthalmologist	☐
	other	☐
If checked:	normal	☐
If abnormal:	abnormal	☐
	referred/ attending ophthalmologist	☐

Criterion 7

Smoking checked in past year?   y☐   n☐   nk☐

	ex-smoker ☐	smoker	☐
If smoker:	advice	☐	
	advice & review	☐	
	smoking clinic	☐	

Criterion 8

BP checked in past year?   y☐   n☐   nk☐

If checked:	normal	☐
	borderline	☐
	raised	☐
If raised:	BP review planned	☐
	start drugs	☐
	alter drugs	☐

Figure 4.1 Data collection form for individual patient

Data collection form

Diabetes protocol

√ = Yes   **x** = No   n = not known   blank = not applicable

| Background data | | | | Must do | | | | | | | | | |
Pat. Code No.	DOB	Sex	Treatment (D-Diet, O-Oral Hypo, I-Insulin, NK-Not known)	1 Patient recorded on diabetic register?	2 Diagnosis correct?	3 Glycated Hb checked in past year? / If yes, result: (normal / abnormal / action taken)	4 Feet checked in past year? / If abnormal, action taken:	5 Urine checked in past year? (Microalbumin / Albumin) / If result +ve, action taken:	6 Fundi checked in past year? / If abnormal, action taken:	7 Smoking checked in past year? / If smoker, action taken:	8 BP checked in last year? / If checked, normal or raised: / If raised, action taken:
TOTALS				TOTALS							TOTALS

Figure 4.2 Data collection form: 10 patients per form

4.2 respectively). If you have a large number of diabetics you may choose to select a random sample (see Chapter 3) for the audit. Identify the patient records from the files and appoint a member of the audit team to extract the relevant data. It is important that another member of the team checks a sample of the forms to verify that data collection is accurate.

Key points

- Diabetes is a common chronic condition which leads to high morbidity and premature mortality.

- Primary care has a key role in the appropriate management of patients with diabetes.

- Prime objectives of long-term systematic monitoring of patients with diabetes are the prevention and/or early detection of complications.

References

American Diabetes Association/National Kidney Foundation (1994). Consensus development conference on the diagnosis and management of nephropathy in patients with diabetes mellitus. *Diabetes Care* **17**: 1357–1361.

Baker, R., Khunti, K. and Lakhani, M. (1993) Audit protocol. In *Monitoring Diabetes*. Leicester: Eli Lilly National Clinical Audit Centre, University of Leicester.

Ballard, D.J., Humphrey, L.L., Melton, J. *et al.* (1988) Epidemiology of persistent proteinuria in Type II diabetes mellitus: population-based study in Rochester, Minnesota. *Diabetes* **37**: 405–412.

Borch-Johnsen, K., Wenzel, H., Viberti, G.C. and Mogensen, C.E. (1993) Is screening and interventions for microalbuminuria worthwhile in patients with insulin dependent diabetes? *BMJ* **306**: 1722–1725.

British Diabetic Association (1993) *Recommendations for the Management of Diabetes in Primary Care*. London: British Diabetic Association.

Clinical Standards Advisory Group (1994) *Standards of Clinical Care for People with Diabetes*. London: HMSO.

Croxon, S.C.M., Burden, A.C., Bodington, M. and Botha, J.L. (1991) The prevalence of diabetes in elderly people. *Diabetic Med.* **8**: 28–31.

Diabetes Control and Complications Trial (DCCT) Research Group (1993) The effect of intensive treatment of diabetes on the development and progression of long term complications in insulin-dependent diabetes mellitus. *N. Engl. J. Med.* **329**: 977–986.

Dierkx, R.I., van de Hoek, W., Hoekstra, J.B. and Erkelens, D.W. (1996) Smoking and diabetes mellitus. *Netherlands J. Med.* **48**: 150–162.

European IDDM Policy Group (1993) Consensus guidelines for the management of insulin-dependent (Type 1) diabetics. *Diabetic Med.* **10**: 990–1005.

Ferris, F.L. (1993) How effective are treatments for diabetic retinopathy? *JAMA* **269**: 1290–1291.

Fuller, J.H. and Stevens, L.K. (1991a) Epidemiology of hypertension in diabetic patients and implications for treatment. *Diabetes Care* **14** (Suppl. 4): 8–12.

Fuller, J.H. and Stevens, L.K. (1991b) Prevalence of hypertension in diabetic patients and its relation to vascular risk. *J. Human Hypertension* **5**: 237–243.

Fuller, J.H. and Head, J. (1989) Blood pressure, proteinuria and their relationship with circulatory mortality: the WHO Multinational Study of Vascular Disease in Diabetes. *Diabetes Metab.* **15**: 273–277.

Gay, E.C., Cai, Y., Gale, S.M. *et al.* (1992) Smokers with IDDM experience excess morbidity. The Colorado IDDM Registry. *Diabetes Care* **15** 947–952.

General Medical Services Committee (1993) *The New Health Promotion Package*. London: British Medical Association.

Greenhalgh, P.M. (1994) *Shared Care for Diabetes: A Systematic Review*. Occasional paper 67. London: Royal College of General Practitioners.

Guidelines Sub-Committee (1993) Guidelines for the management of mild hypertension: memorandum for a World Health Organisation/International Society of Hypertension meeting. *J. Hypertension* **11**: 905–918.

Hawthorne, K., Mello, M. and Tomlinson, S. (1993) Cultural and religious influences in diabetes care in Great Britain. *Diabetic Med.* **10**: 8–12.

Howitt, A.J. and Cheales, N.A. (1993) Diabetes Register: a grass roots approach. *BMJ* **307**: 1046–1048.

Hurwitz, B., Goodman, C. and Yudkin, J. (1993) Prompting the clinical care of non-insulin dependent (Type II) diabetic patients in an inner city area: one model of community care. *BMJ* **306**: 624–630.

Klenerman, L., McCabe, C., Crerand, S. *et al.* (1996) Screening for patients at risk of diabetic foot ulceration in general diabetic outpatient clinic. *Diabetic Med.* **13**: 561–563.

Kohner, E., Allwinkle, J., Andrews, J. *et al.* (1996) Report of the Visual Handicap Group. *Diabetic Med.* **13**: 513–526.

Leese, B. (1991) The cost of diabetes and its complications: a review. York: Centre for Health Economics, University of York.

Litzelmann, D.K., Slemenda, C.W., Langfield, C.D. *et al.* (1993) Reduction of lower extremity clinical abnormalities in patients with non-insulin dependent diabetes mellitus. *Annals Int. Med.* **119**: 36–41.

Malone, J.M., Snyder, M., Anderson, G. *et al.* (1989) Prevention of amputation by diabetic education. *Am. J. Surgery* **158**: 520–523.

Mogensen, C.E., Keane, W.F., Bennett, P.H. *et al.* (1995) Prevention of diabetic renal disease with special reference to microalbuminuria. *Lancet* **346**: 1080–1084.

Most, R.S. and Sinnock, P. (1983) The epidemiology of lower extremity amputations in diabetic individuals. *Diabetes Care* **6**: 87–91.

Paisley, R.B., Macfarlane, D.G., Sherriff, R.J. *et al.* (1980) The relationship between glycosylated and home capillary blood glucose levels in diabetics. *Diabetologia* **19**: 31–34.

Palmberg, P., Smith, M., Waltman, S. *et al.* (1981) The natural history of retinopathy in insulin-dependent juvenile onset diabetes. *Ophthalmology* **88**: 613–618.

Patchett, P. and Roberts, D. (1994) Diabetic patients who do not have diabetes: investigation of register of diabetic patients in general practice. *BMJ*, **308**: 1225–1226.

Pickup, S.C., Crook, M.A. and Tutt, P. (1993) Blood glucose and glycated haemoglobin measurement in hospital: which method? *Diabetic Med.* **10**: 402–411.

St Vincent's Joint Task Force for Diabetes (1995) *The Report*. London: Department of Health and British Diabetic Association.

Tiu, S.C., Lee, S.S. and Cheng, M.W. (1993) Comparison of six commercial techniques in the measurement of microalbuminuria in diabetic patients. *Diabetes Care* **16**: 616–620.

UK Prospective Diabetes Study Group (1990) UK Prospective Diabetes Study VI. Complications of newly diagnosed Type 2 diabetic patients and their association with different clinical and biochemical risk factors. *Diabetes Res.* **13**: 1–11.

Whitford, D.L., Southern, A.J., Braid, E. and Roberts, S.H. (1995) Comprehensive diabetes care in North Tyneside. *Diabetic Med.* **12**: 691–695.

World Health Organisation (Europe) and International Diabetes Federation (Europe) (1990). Diabetes care and research in Europe: the St Vincent's Declaration. *Diabetic Med.* **7**: 360–370.

Yudkin, J.S. (1993) How can we best prolong life? Benefits of coronary risk factor reduction in non-diabetic and diabetic subjects. *BMJ* **306**: 1313–1318.

5

Improving the care of acute illness: a protocol for an audit of patients with acute otitis media

Introduction

Acute otitis media (AOM) is one of the most common reasons for consultation in general practice in the UK – about 30 per cent of British children under 3 years of age see their GP for AOM each year (Ross *et al.*, 1988), of whom 97 per cent receive antibiotics (Froom *et al.*, 1997). Recently there have been calls for a reappraisal of the use of antibiotics for AOM as there is now compelling evidence that routine antibiotic use does not decrease the severity or duration of symptoms nor prevent complications (Del Mar *et al.*, 1997; Froom *et al.*, 1997). There is scope, therefore, for improvement in how AOM is managed in general practice now that authoritative evidence is available to guide management: audit can facilitate this improvement. This chapter describes the development of evidence-based audit criteria for the diagnosis and management of AOM in the setting of UK general practice and their incorporation in an audit protocol.

To identify the elements of care relevant to AOM, we scrutinized one practice guideline developed by the Dutch College of General Practitioners (NHG, 1993), three meta-analyses (Rosenfield *et al.*, 1994; Glasziou *et al.*, 1996; Del Mar *et al.*, 1997) and two review papers (Berman, 1995; Froom *et al.*, 1997). For each identified key element of care further, more detailed, reviews were carried out to identify the strength of evidence prior to developing the criteria.

By this process the following key elements of care were identified: diagnostic criteria for AOM, the appropriate initial management of AOM, indications for antibiotics, the appropriate after-care of patients and the appropriate management of special categories of patients such as those with perforations or repeated episodes of AOM.

Scope

This chapter will concentrate on AOM in children aged 12 or under, as the principal research evidence relates to patients in this age group. The management of patients with otitis media with effusion is specifically excluded.

Audit criteria and their justification

'Must do' criteria

The following have been identified as 'must do' criteria (see Box 5.1).

Box 5.1 Audit criteria for the diagnosis and management of AOM

'Must do' criteria
The records show that:

- The diagnosis of AOM is correct.
- Advice has been given about analgesia.
- Systemic decongestants and/or systemic antihistamines and/or local anaesthetic ear-drops are not prescribed or advised for AOM.
- The first-line antibiotic, if used, is amoxycillin if not contraindicated by allergy.

'Should do' criteria
The records show that:

- When an antibiotic has been prescribed, it is for specific indications, i.e. one or more of the following: persistence of symptoms and/or signs for 48 hours or more; child aged 2 years or under; previous episodes of AOM; failure of conservative treatment; bilateral otitis media; presence of complications.
- A follow up visit has been advised for: (1) patients with a perforated eardrum associated with AOM; (2) patients with a discharging ear within 2–8 weeks after presentation; (3) patients with recurrent AOM within 6 months of presentation.

- *The records show that the diagnosis of AOM is correct*

AOM is often overdiagnosed, as up to 40 per cent of suspected cases may not actually have AOM (Weiss *et al.*, 1996) – this is important as incorrect diagnosis usually leads to unnecessary prescribing of antibiotics. Many of the symptoms and signs of AOM are also seen in children without it (Weiss *et al.*, 1996). Even earache (often due to referred pain) is an inconsistent feature of AOM – in one study less than half the children with earache had AOM (Ingvarsson, 1982). Conversely, AOM can be present without earache (Heikkinen and Ruuskane, 1995). Accordingly, in view of the potential for overdiagnosis, explicit criteria need to be used to diagnose AOM.

AOM has been defined as: 'an infection of the middle ear with an acute onset and duration of less than 3 weeks, characterized by an abnormal eardrum, sometimes accompanied by earache, fever, perforation of the tympanic membrane (TM) or general illness' (NHG 1993). An abnormal eardrum can be defined as 'bulging or opacification of the tympanic membrane with abnormal TM mobility, with or without erythema' (Rosenfield *et al.*, 1994).

Isolated erythema of the eardrum is often the result of a viral infection or crying and should not be the sole basis for diagnosing AOM, since the predictive value of a 'slightly red' TM for AOM is only 16 per cent. In contrast, a cloudy, bulging immobile TM is highly associated with AOM with a predictive value of over 95 per cent (Weiss *et al.*, 1996). AOM is rarely found when the TM is normal (pearly grey, with a light reflex and visible landmarks). The diagnosis of AOM should therefore be based on the findings of a cloudy, bulging TM with or without erythema, or an acute perforation of the TM associated with a discharge (Weiss *et al.*, 1996; NHG, 1993).

In the UK it is common practice to record 'OM' as a shorthand entry in the notes, but this does not allow for a judgement to be made about the basis for the diagnosis. We would recommend, therefore, that a description of the surface of the TM should be recorded along with the configuration of the TM (whether bulging or not), the colour (whether cloudy or not, with or without erythema) and the presence or absence of a perforation.

- *The records show that advice has been given about analgesia*

A major aim of management is to relieve pain and distress. Since the effectiveness of treatments for the pain of AOM has not been studied (Berman, 1995) the optimal management of pain in AOM is uncertain. It is reasonable, however, to recommend standard analgesia such as paracetamol.

- *The records show that systemic decongestants and/or systemic antihistamines and/or local anaesthetic ear-drops are not prescribed or advised for AOM*

There is no place for the use of decongestants and antihistamines as they do not confer benefit (Bain, 1983; Cantekin *et al.*, 1983); they may even cause adverse effects such as nightmares and hallucinations (Sankey *et al.*, 1984). Similarly, topical anaesthetic ear-drops are not recommended (NHG, 1993; anon., 1995).

- *The records show that the first-line antibiotic, if used, is amoxycillin if not contraindicated by allergy*

Numerous reviews have confirmed that if an antibiotic is indicated, the drug of choice is amoxycillin in the absence of allergy (Berman *et al.*, 1997; NHG, 1993; anon., 1995; Rosenfield *et al.*, 1994). Short courses (3 days) are just as effective as long courses in children over the age of 3 years (Bain *et al.*, 1985). This criterion refers to first-line antibiotic treatment. It may be justifiable to use other antibiotics in specific instances such as failure of treatment, or on the basis of culture results, or for some other explicit reason, in which case a record entry should be made to that effect. If the patient is allergic to amoxycillin, then erythromycin should be prescribed (NHG, 1993).

'Should do' criteria

• *The records show that when an antibiotic has been prescribed, it is for one or more of the following specific indications: persistence of symptoms and/or signs for 48 hours or more; child aged 2 years or under; previous episodes of AOM; failure of conservative treatment; bilateral otitis media; presence of complications*

Over 80 per cent of patients with AOM have spontaneous resolution of symptoms and signs (Rosenfield *et al.*, 1994). Although antibiotics reduce pain in a small minority of cases (Rosenfield *et al.*, 1994; Glasziou *et al.*, 1996; Del Mar, 1997), 17 children have to be treated with antibiotics to prevent one child from experiencing pain at 2–7 days after presentation. Antibiotics are also associated with a near doubling of risk of vomiting, diarrhoea or rashes in comparison with placebo. Furthermore, there is no definite evidence of a reduction in complications such as deafness and it is not established whether antibiotics prevent rare complications such as mastoiditis and meningitis.

Unnecessary prescriptions for antibiotics also waste resources and promote the emergence of bacterial resistance (Arason *et al.*, 1996; Froom *et al.*, 1997). The evidence which indicates that routine antibiotic prescribing is unnecessary is supported by experience from the Netherlands where a policy of selective use of antibiotics has been shown to be effective and safe. Complication rates are no higher and rates of bacterial resistance are also reduced (Froom *et al.*, 1997; Van Buchum *et al.*, 1985).

Prescriptions for antibiotics also have the effect of reinforcing the belief amongst patients that they should consult their GP for minor, self-limiting illness (Little *et al.*, 1997). For these reasons antibiotics are not considered to be appropriate *initial* treatment in AOM. Although there is no definite research evidence to identify sub-groups of patients who might benefit from antibiotics from the outset (Majeed and Harris, 1997), there is some evidence from other studies, supported by professional opinion as to which patients ought to be considered for antibiotics (NHG, 1993; Bollag and Bollag-Albrecht, 1991). As this evidence is of a lower level than controlled trials, this criterion is categorized as 'should do'.

In one RCT of children aged 3 years and over, prolonged symptoms occurred on placebo in children with a history of previous OM and bilateral OM, but the differences were small (Burke *et al.*, 1991). Other studies show that children with recurrent AOM are not only less likely to settle spontaneously than those with a first episode of AOM but are also more likely to develop AOM again in the next 12 months (Rasmussen, 1994). Furthermore, children under 2 years are more likely to fail to settle within 48 hours, and poor outcome in AOM is also associated with age under 2 years, bilateral OM and recurrent OM (Jero *et al.*, 1997). Box 5.2 summarizes the indications for antibiotic usage in the management of AOM.

Box 5.2 Indications for antibiotics in AOM

- Age less than 2 years.
- Bilateral otitis media.
- Three or more episodes of AOM in the current year.
- Failed conservative treatment.
- Reattendance within 48 hours.
- Persistent discharging ear.
- Complications, e.g. mastoiditis.
- Down's syndrome, immunocompromised and other high risk patients.

The Dutch guidelines recommend follow-up of patients if antibiotics are not used as initial treatment. Patients aged 2 years and over should be offered follow-up in 3 days if there is no improvement and patients aged 2 years and under in 1 day if there is no improvement.

- *The records show that a follow-up visit has been advised for: (1) patients with a perforated eardrum associated with AOM within 2–8 weeks after presentation; (2) patients with a discharging ear within 2–8 weeks after presentation; (3) patients with recurrent AOM up to 6 months after presentation*

There is great variation in the policies of follow-up intervals of patients after treatment of AOM. Nevertheless, it has been shown that *routine* follow-up of AOM is not needed as parental judgement is a sufficient guide (Hathaway *et al.*, 1994). The Dutch College guidelines recommend follow-up for patients with a perforated eardrum associated with AOM and/or patients with a discharging ear 2–8 weeks after presentation. However, this appears to be a consensus recommendation, as a literature review has failed to find any controlled studies to support this practice. The purpose of follow-up is to ensure that any perforation has healed, since referral is recommended if a perforation persists (NHG standard, 1993; anon., 1995).

Patients with recurrent otitis media are liable to develop otitis media with effusion. Recurrent otitis media is defined as three or more episodes in a year (NHG, 1993) and affected children need careful monitoring for hearing loss. Thus patients with recurrent otitis media should be offered follow-up after an interval of no more than 6 months (Hogan *et al.*, 1997).

Undertaking the audit

Detailed guidance on conducting an audit is given in Chapter 3. Some practices may be able to generate a list of patients with AOM from the practice computer. If this is not possible an encounter form will need to be created on which each doctor in the practice records all cases of AOM over an agreed period of time. The notes can then be extracted and the data collection forms shown can be used (Figures 5.1 and 5.2). According to the total number of patients with AOM a sample may need to be chosen (see Chapter 3).

Data collection form   **Acute otitis media protocol**

Name	
DOB	
Age	
Id No.	

SHOULD DO

Criterion 1
Records contain description
of surface of TM

Colour	y□	n□	dk□
Position	y□	n□	dk□
Perforation	y□	n□	dk□

Diagnosis based on

| Cloudy bulging TM with or without erythema | y□ | n□ | dk□ |
| Perforation with discharge | y□ | n□ | dk□ |

Criterion 2
Advice/prescription for

| analgesia | y□ | n□ | dk□ |

Criterion 3
The following prescribed/advised

Oral decongestants	y□	n□	dk□
Oral antihistamines	y□	n□	dk□
Local anaesthetic ear-drops	y□	n□	dk□

Criterion 4
If antibiotics used was it

| Amoxycillin | y□ | n□ | dk□ |
| If no, reason stated | y□ | n□ | |

Criterion 5
Indications for antibiotic if used

Persistence of symptoms/ signs	y□	n□	dk□
Child aged ⩽ 2	y□	n□	dk□
Previous AOM	y□	n□	dk□
Failure of conservative treatment	y□	n□	dk□
Bilateral OM	y□	n□	dk□
Complications	y□	n□	dk□
None of the above	y□	n□	dk□

Criterion 6
Follow-up offered/taken place

Perforated eardrum	y□	n□	dk□
Discharging ear	y□	n□	dk□
Recurrent AOM	y□	n□	dk□

Figure 5.1 Data collection form for individual patient

Data collection form

Practice code

√ = Yes, ✗ = No, O = DK

Acute otitis media protocol

Patient initials or code	Age	Sex	Diagnosis correct: cloudy, bulging TM or perforation	Analgesia advised/ prescribed	Inappropriate prescribing			Antibiotic used, amoxycillin	Specified indication for antibiotic (Criterion 5)	Should do		
					Oral decongestants	Oral antihistamines	Topical anaesthetic ear-drops			Follow-up		
										Perforated eardrum	Discharge	Recurrent AOM
TOTALS										TOTALS		

Figure 5.2 Data collection form: 10 patients per form

Key points

- AOM is frequently overdiagnosed; the diagnosis should only be made in the presence of a cloudy, bulging TM with or without erythema or an acute perforation of the TM with a discharge.

- AOM must not be diagnosed if the eardrum is normal or shows erythema only.

- Antibiotics are not routinely indicated as initial treatment in AOM.

- When an antibiotic is indicated, amoxycillin should be the first-line choice.

- Routine follow-up should only be initiated for patients with a perforated eardrum and/or recurrent AOM; it is not necessary for the vast majority of patients with AOM.

References

Anon. (1995) Management of acute otitis media and glue ear. *Drug and Therapeutics Bulletin* **33**: 12–15.

Arason, V.A., Kristinsson, K.G., Sigurdsson, J.A. *et al.* (1996) Do antimicrobials increase the carriage rate of penicillin resistant pneumococci in children? Cross sectional study. *BMJ* **313**: 3887–3891.

Bain, D.J.G. (1983) Can the clinical course of acute otitis media be modified by systemic decongestant or antihistamine treatment? *BMJ* **287**: 654–656.

Bain, D.J.G., Murphy, E. and Ross, F. (1985). Acute otitis media: clinical course among children who received a short course of high dose antibiotic. *BMJ* **291**: 1243–1246.

Berman, S. (1995) Otitis media in children. *N. Engl. J. Med.* **332**: 1560–1565.

Berman, S., Byrns, P.J., Bondy, T. *et al.* (1997) Otitis media related antibiotic prescribing patterns, outcomes and expenditures. *Pediatrics* **100 (4)**: 585–592.

Bollag, U. and Bollag-Albrecht, E. (1991) Recommendations derived from practice audit for the treatment of acute otitis media. *Lancet* **338**: 96–99.

Burke, P., Bain, J., Robinson, D. *et al.* (1991) Acute red ear in children: controlled trial of non-antibiotic treatment in general practice. *BMJ* **303**: 558-562.

Cantekin, E.I., Mandell, E.M., Bluestone, C.D. *et al.* (1983) Lack of efficacy of a decongestant-antihistamine combination for otitis media in children. *N. Engl. J. Med.* **308**: 297–301.

Del Mar, D., Glasziou, P. and Hayem, M. (1987) Are antibiotics indicated as initial treatment for children with acute otitis media? A meta-analysis. *BMJ* **314**: 1526–1529.

Froom, J., Culpepper, L., de Melker, R. *et al.* (1997) Antimicrobials for acute otitis media? A review from the International Primary Care Network. *BMJ* **315**: 98–102.

Glasziou, P., Hayem, M. and Del Mar, C.B. (1996) Treatments for acute otitis media in children: antibiotic versus placebo. In *Respiratory Infections Module of the Cochrane Database of Systematic Reviews*. (Eds Douglas, R., Berman, S., Black, R.E. *et al.*). Oxford: Update Software.

Hathaway, T.J., Katz, H.P., Dershewitz, R.A. *et al.* (1994) Acute otitis media: who needs post treatment follow up. *Pediatrics* **94**: 143–147.

Heikkinen, T. and Ruuskane, O. (1995) Signs and symptoms predicting acute otitis media. *Arch. Pediatr. Adolesc.* **149** (1): 26–29.

Hogan, S.C., Stratford, K.J. and Moore, D.C. (1997) Duration and recurrence of otitis media with effusion in children from birth to 3 years. *BMJ* **314**: 350–355

Ingvarsson, L. (1982) Acute otalgia in children – findings and diagnosis. *Acta Paediatr. Scand.* **71**: 705–710.

Jero, J., Virolainen, A., Virtanen, M. *et al.* (1997) Prognosis of acute otitis media: factors associated with poor outcome. *Acta Oto-laryngologica* **117**: 278–283.

Little, P., Williamson, I., Warner, G. *et al.* (1997) Open randomised trial of prescribing strategies in managing sore throat. *BMJ* **414**: 722–727.

Majeed, A. and Harris, T. (1997) Acute otitis media in children. *BMJ* **7**: 323–324.

NHG (1993) Dutch College of General Practitioners standard for acute otitis media. Utrecht: NHG.

Rasmussen, F. (1994) Recurrence of acute otitis media at pre-school age in Sweden. *J Epidemiol. Community Health* **48**: 33–35.

Rosenfield, R., Vertrees, J., Carr, J. *et al.* (1994) Clinical efficacy of antimicrobial drugs for acute otitis media: a meta-analysis of 5400 children from thirty-three randomised trials. *J. Pediatrics* **124**: 355–367.

Ross, A.K., Croft, P.R. and Collins, M. (1988) Incidence of acute otitis media in infants in a general practice. *J. Roy. Coll. Gen. Pract.* **38**: 70–72.

Sankey, R., Nunn, A. and Sills, J. (1984) Visual hallucinations in children receiving decongestants. *BMJ* **288**: 1369.

Van Buchem, F.L., Peeters, M.F. and van't Hof, M.A. (1985) Acute otitis media: a new treatment strategy. *BMJ* **290**: 1033–1037.

Weiss, J.C., Yates, G.R. and Quinn, L.D. (1996) Acute otitis media. Making an accurate diagnosis. *Am. Family Physician* **53**: 1200–1206.

6

Improving practice organization: a protocol for an audit of patients' routine access to their general practitioner

Introduction

In this chapter we will describe the development of an audit protocol related to patient access to general practice. For most patients general practice is the first point of contact with organized medical services and patients themselves make the initial decision whether or not to consult. 'Unfortunately for doctors, the decision to seek medical care does *not* occur at a uniformly recognized and predictable threshold, nor does it correlate closely with the potential seriousness of the symptoms experienced by a patient' (Fraser, 1992). Consequently, as doctors of first contact, GPs have an obligation to ensure that patients have ready access to them so that an initial decision about their health status can be taken without undue delay.

Furthermore, surveys have repeatedly shown that patients attach great importance to the need for easy accessibility to their GP. For example, in one study patients expressed dissatisfaction with receptionists and appointment systems (Cartwright and Anderson, 1981) and in another were critical of perceived lack of availability of appointments (Leavey, 1985). In a more recent study of satisfaction involving 17 000 patients, the availability of appointments was one of the most poorly rated aspects of general practice (Baker and Streatfield, 1996), and in a consumer survey it was established that patients particularly wanted improved appointment access, shorter waiting times, longer consultation times, continuity and helpful receptionists (*Which?*, 1995).

Scope

Although a variety of approaches could be adopted, it was our intention to develop an audit protocol relating to the routine access of patients to their GP during normal working hours. Therefore, associated topics such as out of hours care and home visits were excluded, as the types of patients involved and the issues of concern are sufficiently different to make these topics for separate audits. Since we were concerned with the availability of appointments rather than the interpersonal skills of receptionists who operate appointment systems, consideration of the performance of receptionists was also excluded.

To identify the elements of care relevant to obtaining access, we undertook a search for reviews and guidelines concerned with access to general practice. We found no relevant guidelines, although there were some reviews which were used to identify the key elements of care relevant to UK general practice (see Box 6.1).

Box 6.1 The identified key elements of care

- Availability of appointments, including wait for appointments and flexibility of the appointment system in catering for more urgent cases and those people who have difficulties with appointment systems.
- Length of appointments.
- Telephone access to GPs.
- Continuity of care.
- Opening hours.
- Waiting room times.
- Comprehensiveness of services.

Some other identified elements of care were excluded as they were less relevant (length of appointments, opening hours and comprehensiveness of services). Although appointment length is an issue that had been investigated in several studies, it is not directly related to the topic of accessibility, but becomes important once access has been obtained. Practice opening hours can be important to some patients, and a practice might consider undertaking a patient survey to discover whether different opening hours would be preferred. However, we decided to exclude this element of care because most practices are unlikely to be able to make substantial changes in their opening hours, and relatively little research has been undertaken on this topic. For the majority of practices, it would be more important to make best use of existing opening hours to ensure convenient patient access.

Many health care teams offer a comprehensive range of services provided by practice nurses, counsellors, physiotherapists, health visitors and other health professionals. Although access to these professionals may be important for many patients, the scope of the audit had been defined as access to GPs. Therefore, access to other professionals was excluded.

Audit criteria and their justification

For each element of care, more detailed additional reviews were undertaken to identify the strength of research evidence and to facilitate the development of criteria (see Box 6.2). Each criterion is followed by an explanation as to why it has been classified as 'must do' or 'should do'.

Box 6.2 Audit criteria

'Must do' criteria
- Patients who request a same day appointment with a GP are offered an appointment on the same day or speak directly to a GP in the practice.
- Patients who request a routine appointment are able to see the doctor of their choice.

'Should do' criteria
- Patients who request an appointment but state that they do not need the appointment on the same day are able to see a doctor in not more than 3 working days.
- The wait between the allocated appointment time and the start of a consultation is not more than 20 minutes.
- The practice should have a system to enable patients to speak to a GP by telephone and the arrangements for contacting the GP should be publicized to patients.

'Must do' criteria

- *Patients who request a same day appointment with a GP are offered an appointment on the same day or speak directly to a GP in the practice*

There are no RCTs of different responses to requests for same day appointments. However, the arguments for rapid access to care for those patients who believe they have an urgent medical problem are such as to make ethical approval for a trial unlikely.

The level of agreement about the importance of access to care is evident in recommendations from regulatory agencies. Guidance from the General Medical Council on good medical practice includes advice to doctors to take suitable and prompt action when necessary (GMC, 1995). The terms of service for GPs also state that: 'The doctor will normally be available at such times and places as shall have been approved by the health authority, and will inform patients about this availability' [The National Health Service (General Medical Services) Regulations, 1992]. In addition, the Medical Defence Union points out that: 'A flexible system for both routine and urgent appointments is helpful and may limit frustration on initial contact with the practice' (Green *et al.*, 1996).

Despite this advice, patients do report difficulties in obtaining appointments. In a survey of over 1000 adults, 58 per cent said that is was difficult or impossible to get an appointment to see their own doctor on the same day (Arber and Sawyer, 1981). It is likely that some requests for same day appointments are not justifiable in terms of medical need, although they may be in terms of patient convenience. However, in a study in one practice patients who asked to be given an appointment on the same day were compared to those who asked for routine appointments (Field, 1980). Those requesting appointments on the same day generally had good clinical reasons for their requests, and did not appear to be abusing the system. Another reason for offering rapid access to care in addition to clinical need is that some patients may find appointment systems confusing and difficult to use. For example, among patient factors related to defaulting from appointments are psychological problems and higher consultation rates (Cosgrove, 1990). In a study in a practice serving a deprived population, patients attending without appointments were more likely to be single parents or lack other social support (Virji, 1990). In consequence it was suggested that practices serving deprived communities should consider providing mixed open access and appointment systems.

It has been demonstrated in one practice that it is possible to offer appointments on the same day to 98 per cent of those patients who make this request (Fishbacher and Robertson, 1986). In another study of 641 patients, 90 per cent of those requesting an urgent appointment reported seeing the doctor on the same day (Allen *et al.*, 1988). Practices may use a variety of methods to ensure that patients can be seen quickly. In some, all appointments are prebookable, with 'urgent' patients being fitted in as extras (Eve *et al.*, 1996). Others reserve a proportion of appointments for booking on the same day, or provide open surgery sessions each day with one or more 'duty' doctors. One practice chose to run 'open-ended' morning consulting sessions for each GP, and reported a decline in evening appointments and a low rate of home visits (Greig, 1984).

In summary, this criterion was categorized as 'must do' because professional organizations and health service regulations accept that patients with acute illness or symptoms suggesting potentially serious conditions must be able to see a doctor quickly. There are no RCTs to test this belief, but such trials would be virtually impossible to justify. Furthermore, on most occasions, patients' demands for same day appointments can be met and are mostly justifiable.

- *Patients who request a routine appointment are able to see the doctor of their choice*

There is considerable evidence about the importance to patients of continuity of care. Higher levels of continuity are consistently associated with higher levels of patient satisfaction (Hjortdahl and Laerum, 1992; Linn *et al.*, 1985; Baker and Whitfield, 1992), and being able to see the same doctor has been rated by patients as being one of the more important features of general practice (Smith and Armstrong, 1988). Nevertheless, continuity is less important to some patients than ease of access and choice. Furthermore, 68 per cent of practice patients requesting a non-urgent appointment expressed a preference for a particular doctor or time (Fishbacher and Robertson, 1986), and female patients have a preference for a female doctor when consulting for gynaecological problems (Preston-Whyte *et al.*, 1983). In summary, our recommendation is that continuity should be offered to patients but appointment systems should be sufficiently flexible to accommodate patients who prefer quick access to any doctor in the practice.

'Should do' criteria

The following criteria have been classified as 'should do'.

• *Patients who request an appointment but state that they do not need the appointment on the same day are able to see a doctor in not more than 3 working days*

There is good evidence that many patients are dissatisfied with the availability of routine appointments. In a study involving 99 practices and 17 799 patients, availability was the aspect of care which attracted the lowest rating (Baker, 1996). In approximately one third of the practices, ratings of satisfaction with availability were below 50 per cent. Cartwright and Anderson (1981) reported that 33 per cent of patients regarded the delay for appointments as unreasonable if they had to wait between 1 and 3 days, with 71 per cent feeling that a wait of more than 3 days was unreasonable. 40 per cent of patients who had to wait longer than 3 days said this had caused them not to see their doctor on some occasion in the previous 12 months. The proportion of patients who fail to attend their appointments increases as the number of days between the appointment and its booking increases, and efficient appointment systems may reduce the number of defaulters (Bickler, 1985).

There is wide variation between different practices in consultation rates and the numbers of appointments offered. In a study involving 26 Scottish practices, the consultation rate varied from 2.24 to 5.98 per patient per year (McRae and Foster, 1996). The number of appointments offered by the practices also varied from 30 to 104 per 1000 patients per week, and 'extras' from 0.75 to 19.8 per 1000 per week. The findings indicate that practices could reduce the numbers of 'extras' by increasing the total number of appointments, provided the total consultation rate was not more than 75 per 1000 patients per week. In those practices that were particularly busy and had to provide more than this number of consultations to meet patient demand, increasing the number of bookable appointments appeared to have no impact on the number of extras. Thus, practices in areas of high demand face particular problems in designing their appointments systems.

However, for most practices, appointment systems can be organized to permit access within 3 days for most patients. Indeed, in the survey of Allen *et al.* (1988), 78 per cent of patients reported being able to see the doctor of their choice within 2 working days. Individual practices have reported that changes to appointment systems can reduce delays for appointments, for example by increasing the number of appointments bookable in advance (Baker, 1990). A computerized appointment system can improve efficiency by reducing the time required to book an appointment by telephone or in person (Campbell *et al.*, 1996).

In summary, this criterion has been categorized as 'should do' because there is consistent evidence that patients want short delays for appointments, and that satisfaction declines steeply when delays

are longer than 3 days. Most practices are able to meet this requirement, although some in underprivileged areas with highly demanding
patients may find this impossible. However, there are no RCTs which
compare the impact of short and long delays on patient outcome.
Therefore categorization as 'must do' could not be justified.

- *The wait between the allocated appointment time and the start of a
  consultation is not more than 20 minutes*

The relationship between appointment booking interval and patient
waiting times has been demonstrated through mathematical model-
ling (Hill-Smith, 1989). An appointment interval which is less than
the actual median consultation length results in long waits for
patients. Patients dislike long waits between their appointment time
and their actual consultation. Twelve per cent of patients found a wait
of more than 20 minutes unreasonable, 34 per cent found a wait of
30 or more minutes unreasonable, and 50 per cent thought a wait of
45 minutes or longer unreasonable (Cartwright and Anderson 1979).
In a study involving over 6000 patients, 63 per cent were seen within
a waiting time of 14 minutes, but 33 per cent had to wait between 15
and 40 minutes (Heaney *et al.*, 1991). The proportion of dissatisfied
patients increased from 20 per cent of those who waited 15–29 minutes to 50 per cent of those waiting 30–44 minutes. Patients seen at
the end of consultation sessions tend to have to wait longer than
those seen at the start.

Several audits have shown that practices can implement changes to
reduce waiting times. In one practice, the proportion of patients waiting over 30 minutes was reduced from 11 per cent to 7 per cent
(Davies *et al.*, 1995). Another practice reduced patient waiting time
by introducing a small increase in consultation booking intervals
(MacFarland and Armstrong, 1995). A flexible system in which
patients choose the length of their appointment booking can be
another appropriate alternative (Harrison, 1988).

In summary, this criterion was categorized as 'should do' because
long waiting times lead to patient dissatisfaction and it is possible to
design appointment systems to avoid long waits on most occasions.
However, there are no RCTs of the impact of different waiting times,
and categorization as 'must do' was not justified.

- *The practice should have a system to enable patients to speak to a GP
  by telephone and the arrangements for contacting the GP should be
  publicized to patients*

Most GPs accept non-emergency telephone calls from patients during the day (Hallam, 1991). In this survey, some GPs reported setting
aside specific times for receiving calls, although the majority received
fewer than four calls per day. Among doctors who received a mean of
nine or more calls per day, telephone advice about current illnesses
was accompanied by instructions to attend surgery if symptoms did
not resolve (Hallam, 1992). However, some groups of patients may
find telephone advice an unsatisfactory alternative to consultations,
for example Asian patients (Rashid and Jagger, 1992).

Patients do encounter difficulties in being able to contact their general practice by telephone. Indeed, in one study, over half the patients were unable to get through to the practice on the first attempt, although when patients were able to speak to doctors on the telephone, satisfaction was high (Hallam, 1993). It was suggested that practices should have one incoming telephone line per 2500 patients. In one practice, patients reported that the practice telephone line was engaged for 57 per cent of first calls (Marshall, 1993), whilst in another, 80 per cent of callers were able to get through at the first attempt (Child, 1995).

The medical lists of health authorities are required to include the telephone numbers at which every GP is prepared to receive messages [The National Health Service (General Medical Services) Regulations, 1992]. Even so, many patients are unaware that their practice has a policy on patient telephone access to GPs (Hallam, 1993).

In summary, this criterion was included because patients appreciate telephone access, and GPs can find this an efficient contribution to patient care. However, patients do not always know about arrangements for telephone access and therefore practices should provide this information.

Undertaking the audit

The criteria in this audit require that three different methods of collecting data are used. Data for the first three criteria can be collected as patients request appointments. Information about waits for appointments must be collected by a different system in which doctors record the start time for each consultation. The final criterion concerns systems to enable patients to speak to a GP by telephone. For the audit, all that is required is to check that the practice has such a system. These three methods of data collection are discussed below.

Collecting data about appointments

The first three criteria are concerned with patients' requests for appointments with a GP. Although clinical records are the most common source of data for audit, they cannot be used for this topic. Therefore, a specific data collection form is required (see Figure 6.1). Copies of the form must be available to any member of staff who may be required to respond to requests for appointments. For convenience, it would be sensible for the forms to be located near the appointment book or computer terminals used to book appointments. Appointments requested by telephone or in person must also be included. Because these forms are completed as patients request appointments, they are sometimes referred to as 'encounter forms'.

Date:				Form number:		
Patient number	Appointment request by 1 = tel. 2 = in person	Same day requested? 1 = yes 2 = no	Given same day appointment 1 = yes 2 = no	Spoken to GP 1 = yes 2 = no	GP of choice 1 = yes 2 = no	Days to appointment

Figure 6.1 Encounter form for collecting data about appointments

The encounter form captures information relating to the first three criteria. As patients request appointments, they should be allocated an identification number (which practices may choose to cross-reference with the name in the appointment book). The other columns are self-explanatory and information about the appointment should be entered as appropriate, using the numbers 1 or 2 as required. The wait from request to actual appointment is calculated in working days with Saturdays excluded if the practice does not hold routine appointments on Saturdays.

The findings may be influenced by coincidental factors. For example, if one GP is on holiday, or if there is an influenza epidemic there would be particular pressure on the appointment system. Therefore, the data collection period should be chosen to avoid such factors. Furthermore, data collection should be for a sufficiently long period to ensure that an adequate number of patients is included. Shorter data collection periods will also be at greater risk of influence by special circumstances. Therefore, we recommend the selection of a random number of working days over a period of 2 months. Fifteen days should be included, with data being collected about every appointment request on those days. The days can be selected by allocating a number to each day in advance and then using a table of random numbers to identify which ones should be included (see Chapter 3 for advice on taking a random sample).

Waiting for consultations

Figure 6.2 shows an example of a recording form which can capture the information on the length of time patients wait for their consultations. Each GP on the days chosen for data collection should complete such a form throughout each consulting session. It may be helpful to provide all included GPs with a small desk clock, with the time of each clock being used in the audit synchronized.

Every GP at the practice should take part. Both morning and evening consulting sessions must be included, and we recommend at least 10 sessions for each GP. If possible, these 10 sessions should be selected at random from a larger number of sessions over a period such as 2 months.

Patient	Booked appointment time	Actual start time	Wait (minutes)	Wait within 20 minutes? 1 = yes 2 = no

Figure 6.2 Appointment waiting time recording form

Arrangements for telephoning the GP

The practice either does or does not have arrangements for telephone access, and does or does not publish relevant information to patients. No formal data collection is required.

Key points

- Patients place a high priority on easy access to GPs.
- Continuity of care with a particular GP is also important to many patients.
- Effective strategies for providing rapid access and continuity suitable for most practices are available.
- Prospective audit of patient access is easy to conduct.

References

Allen, D., Leavey, R. and Marks, B. (1988) Survey of patients' satisfaction with access to general practitioners. *J. Roy. Coll. Gen. Pract.* **38**: 163–165.

Arber, S. and Sawyer, L. (1981) Changes in general practice: do patients benefit? *BMJ* **283**: 1367–1370.

Baker, R. (1996) The measurement of patient satisfaction in general practice. MD Thesis, University of London.

Baker, R. (1990) Problem solving with audits in general practice. *BMJ* **300**: 378–380.

Baker, R. and Streatfield, J. (1995) What type of practice do patients prefer? Exploration of practice characteristics influencing patient satisfaction. *Br. J. Gen. Pract.* **45**: 654–659.

Baker, R. and Whitfield, M. (1992) Measuring patient satisfaction: a test of construct validity. *Quality in Health Care* **1**: 104–109.

Bickler, C.B. (1985) Defaulted appointments in general practice. *J. Roy. Coll. Gen. Pract.* **35**: 19–22.

Campbell, S.M., Roland, M.O. and Gormanly, B. (1996) Evaluation of a computerised appointment system in general practice. *Br. J. Gen. Pract.* **46**: 477–478.

Cartwright, A. and Anderson, R. (1979) *Patients and their doctors 1977.* Occasional paper 8. London: Royal College of General Practitioners.

Cartwright, A. and Anderson, R. (1981) *General Practice Revisited. A second study of patients and their doctors.* London: Tavistock Publications.

Child, D. (1995) Access by telephone. *Audit in General Practice* **3** (2): 11–12.

Cosgrove, M.P. (1990) Defaulters in general practice: reasons for default patterns of attendance. *Br. J. Gen. Pract.* **40**: 50–52

Davies, H.M., Williams, D.K., Davies, D.W. *et al.* (1995) Are people satisfied with the service we provide? *Audit in General Practice* **3** (2): 20–22.

Eve, R., Waller, J., Jenkins, P. and McGorrigan, J. (1996) *When is your next appointment? An exploration of general practice appointment systems.* Sheffield: Towards co-ordinated practice. Sheffield Health Authority.

Field, J. (1980) Problems of urgent consultations within an appointment system. *J. Roy. Coll. Gen. Pract.* **30**: 173–177.

Fishbacher, C.M. and Robertson, R.A. (1986) Patients' difficulties in obtaining appointments – a general practice audit. *J. Roy. Coll. Gen. Pract.* **36**: 282–284.

Fraser, R.C. (1992) Setting the scene. In *Clinical Method. A General Practice Approach*, 2nd Edn (Ed. Fraser, R.C.). Oxford: Butterworth-Heinemann.

GMC (1995) Good medical practice. Guidance from the General Medical Council. London: GMC.

Green, S., Goodwin, H. and Moss, J. (1996) *Problems in General Practice. Complaints and How to Avoid Them.* London: Medical Defence Union.

Greig, D.N.H. (1984) Making an appointment system work. *BMJ* **288**: 1423–1425.

Hallam, L. (1991) Organisation of telephone services and patients' access to doctors by telephone in general practice. *BMJ* **302**: 629–632.

Hallam, L. (1992) Patient access to GPs by telephone: the doctor's view. *Br. J. Gen. Pract.* **42**: 186–189.

Hallam, L. (1993) Access to general practice and GPs by telephone: the patients' view. *Br. J. Gen. Pract.* **43**: 331–335.

Harrison, A.T. (1988) Appointment systems: evaluation of a flexible system offering patients limited choice. *BMJ* **296**: 685–686.

Heaney, D.J., Howie, J.G.R. and Porter, A.M.D. (1991) Factors influencing waiting times and consultation times in general practice. *Br. J. Gen. Pract.* **41**: 315–319.

Hill-Smith, I. (1989) Mathematical relationship between waiting times and appointment interval for doctor and patients. *J. Roy. Coll. Gen. Pract.* **39**: 492–494.

Hjortdahl, P. and Laerum, E. (1992) Continuity of care in general practice: effect on patient satisfaction. *BMJ* **304**: 1287–1290.

Leavey, R. (1985) Access to GPs: a fair share for all. A report for the DHSS. Manchester: Manchester Centre for Primary Care Research.

Linn, L.S., Brook, R.H., Clark, V.A. *et al.* (1985) Physician and patient satisfaction factors related to the organization of internal medicine group practices. *Medical Care* **23**: 1171–1178.

MacFarland, J.R. and Armstrong, K.J. (1995) More waiting time for patients, less waiting around. *Audit in General Practice* **3** (4): 14–17.

Marshall, M.N. (1993) Telephone access in general practice. *Br. J. Gen. Pract.* **43**: 535–536.

McRae, F. and Foster, J. (1996) Availability of appointments. In Lothian Audit Packages, second report 1992/94, pp. 49–71. Edinburgh: Edinburgh Healthcare Trust.

Preston-Whyte, M.E., Fraser, R.C. and Beckett, J.L. (1983) The effect of a principal's gender on consultation patterns in general practice. *J. Roy. Coll. Gen. Pract.* **33**: 654–658.

Rashid, A. and Jagger, C. (1992) Attitudes to and perceived use of health care services among Asian and non-Asian patients in Leicester. *Br. J. Gen. Pract.* **42**: 197–201.

Smith, C.H. and Armstrong, D. (1989) Comparison of criteria derived by government and patients for evaluating GP services. *BMJ* **299**: 494–496.

The National Health Service (General Medical Services) Regulations 1992. Terms of Service for Doctors (Schedule 2, paragraph 29). London: HMSO.

Virji, A. (1990) A study of patients attending without appointments in an urban general practice. *BMJ* **301**: 22–26

Which? (1995) What makes a good GP? *Which?* June 18.

7

Improving health promotion activity: a protocol for an audit of helping patients to stop smoking

Introduction

Earlier chapters deal with audit of clinical and organizational topics in primary care. In this chapter we describe how the principles outlined in Chapters 1–3 should be used to audit a health promotion topic: the management of smoking cessation. Although some GPs find health promotion boring (Williams and Calnan, 1994), GPs can be highly effective in helping patients to stop smoking (Ashenden *et al.*, 1997). Nevertheless, considerable negotiating skills are needed. Accordingly, helping patients to stop smoking is a challenging task which should be undertaken by all GPs. In this chapter, we will illustrate how GPs' attempts to help patients stop smoking can be effectively audited.

Although population smoking rates have declined in recent years, 29 per cent of men and 27 per cent of women in the UK still smoked in 1992 (Office of Population Censuses and Surveys, 1994). Smoking causes much morbidity and many fatal diseases (Doll and Peto, 1976), and smoking-related illness costs the NHS around £611 million annually (Health Education Authority, 1991). Clearly smoking tobacco remains an enormous public health problem which requires an appropriate response from all clinicians when encountering patients who smoke.

One intervention which would help address the major health threat posed by smoking is to conduct effective audit of the primary care management of smokers. Smoking satisfies all the requirements for audit because, in addition to the above, there is compelling evidence that GPs can promote smoking cessation in patients (Silagy *et al.*, 1997). Furthermore, since GPs do not routinely deliver anti-smoking intervention, opportunities exist for substantial improvement in this area of clinical practice (Silagy *et al.*, 1992; Coleman and Wilson, 1996).

There is an extensive literature on the subject of smoking cessation in primary care, including an evidence-based guideline (Fiore *et al.*,

1996) and many high quality RCTs of interventions. The research evidence identifies four key elements of care. Firstly, it is essential that information on patients' smoking habits is regularly ascertained and documented. Secondly, it is essential to determine smokers' motivation to stop. Thirdly, simple, effective anti-smoking interventions are available which can be easily used by GPs. These include brief advice, leaflets and nicotine replacement therapy (NRT). Fourthly, providing reinforcement of interventions is important as this increases the success rates of smokers who try to stop. We have used these key elements to produce audit criteria that are relevant and feasible for use in primary care. Conducting an audit which increases compliance with these criteria will, therefore, enhance the primary care management of smoking and help alleviate a major public health problem.

Scope

This audit is restricted to dealing with adult patients because little work has been done to determine whether primary care anti-smoking interventions are effective with teenagers and children. The audit criteria described in the next section are suitable for:

- all types of tobacco smoking;
- adult men and women (aged 16 or over).

Figure 7.1 summarizes the key elements in the primary care management of smoking cessation and indicates how compliance with our audit criteria (shown in italics) ensures that key elements of care are addressed. The audit criteria (Box 7.1) have been explicitly related to patient attendance to encourage the incorporation of opportunistic anti-smoking interventions into routine clinical practice. There are five criteria and all are 'must do'. The following section explains the reasoning behind the development of each criterion.

Box 7.1   Audit criteria

'Must do' criteria

For smokers who have consulted in the past 12 months the records show that:

- At least annually, the smoking status of the patient and the number of cigarettes smoked daily have been recorded.
- At least annually, the smoker's motivation to stop has been ascertained.
- At least annually, smoking cessation has been discussed and those motivated to stop are offered a follow-up consultation.
- At least annually, motivated patients who smoke more than 10 cigarettes a day have been recommended to use nicotine replacement therapy.
- Pregnant smokers have had smoking cessation discussed with them and those motivated to stop are offered a follow-up consultation.

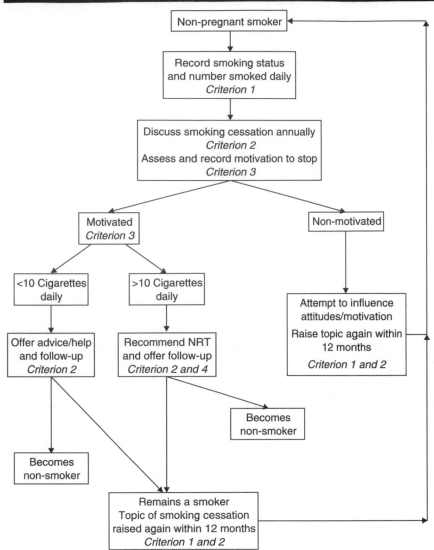

Figure 7.1 Key elements in the management of smoking cessation

Audit criteria and their justification

'Must do' criteria

- *For smokers who have consulted in the past 12 months the records show that, at least annually, the smoking status of the patient and the number of cigarettes smoked daily have been recorded*

Box 7.2 gives details of how to define whether or not a patient is a smoker. Anyone who has smoked a cigarette within the last 4 months should be considered for inclusion in the audit. It is reasonable to classify as ex-smokers those who have stopped smoking for 4 months or longer because most smokers who manage to stop for 4 months will not restart (Marlatt *et al.*, 1988). This definition allows the inclusion of occasional smokers and smokers who are currently attempting to stop, as advice given to smokers who are trying to stop is likely to be most effective (Di Clemente *et al.*, 1991).

Having a systematic approach towards documenting patients' smoking status increases the frequency with which doctors advise against smoking (Fiore *et al.*, 1996). As this is a key element in the management of smoking cessation, this criterion was categorized as 'must do'.

Box 7.2   Smoking behaviour: definitions

- Smoker: someone having smoked tobacco in the previous 4 months.
- Non-smoker: someone who has never smoked.
- Ex-smoker: someone who has not smoked for at least 4 months.

Since only those who smoke more than 10 cigarettes daily will benefit from NRT (Silagy *et al.*, 1997) it is essential to determine the number of cigarettes smoked daily. Consequently this part of the criterion is also categorized as 'must do'.

Clinicians need to return to the topic of smoking with those who do not attempt to stop or who unsuccessfully attempt cessation. There is no evidence to suggest the optimum period before raising the topic again, but annual enquiry about smoking status and the quantity smoked will keep smoking firmly on the clinical agenda. The recording of smoking status and any discussion about smoking have been deliberately separated to prevent confusion between these two issues.

- *For smokers who have consulted in the past 12 months the records show that, at least annually, smoking cessation has been discussed and those motivated to stop are offered a follow-up consultation*

Discussing smoking. After receiving brief advice against smoking from GPs, approximately two out of every 50 smokers will stop within one year (Kottke *et al.*, 1988. Silagy and Ketteridge, 1996; Ashenden *et al.*, 1997). Since GPs have higher contact rates with patients, it is sensible to recommend that they initially give advice, and as the provision of advice against smoking has a direct effect on patients' smoking rates this is a 'must do' criterion.

Nature of advice. There is insufficient research evidence to enable recommendations to be made about the type of advice which would be most effective. UK studies have allowed participating GPs to give advice against smoking in their own style, but the actual content of advice has never been monitored (Russell *et al.*, 1979, 1983; Jamrozik *et al.*, 1984). Anti-smoking leaflets can have an independent effect on motivated smokers in the absence of advice to stop: where leaflets are given to smokers who agree that they want to stop, one in 50 will do so (Slama *et al.*, 1995). Leaflets can also reinforce the effects of GPs' advice against smoking when it is given (Russell *et al.*, 1979). Consequently we suggest that *any discussion where smoking is mentioned, and it is made clear to the smoker that their habit is undesirable*, is recorded as the smoker having been advised.

Follow-up. The greater contact smokers have with those advising them against smoking, the more likely they are to stop (Kottke *et al.*, 1988; Silagy and Ketteridge, 1996; Ashenden *et al.*, 1997). It is unimportant *which* primary health care team member provides the follow-up consultation, as it has been shown that repeated, consistent advice is effective, irrespective of the status of the health care professional who delivers this (Kottke *et al.*, 1988). As reinforcement of anti-smoking advice by providing follow-up increases the efficacy of advice, this criterion is a 'must do'.

- *For smokers who have consulted in the last 12 months the records show that, at least annually, the smoker's motivation to stop has been ascertained*

Unfortunately, there is no universally accepted method for assessing a smoker's motivation to stop. For audit purposes, a simple approach is to define *motivated* smokers as those who state that they want to stop (Slama *et al.*, 1995).

Motivated smokers using NRT are much more likely to manage to stop (Silagy *et al.*, 1997), and those who stop for at least 1 week have a one in four chance of not smoking for at least 1 year (Yudkin *et al.*, 1996). In smokers for whom NRT is not recommended (less than 10 cigarettes daily), motivation is also important. Greater motivation to stop is associated with making more smoking cessation attempts (Marsh and Matheson, 1983; Jackson *et al.*, 1986; Di Clemente *et al.*, 1991). As motivation is a quality which has a direct effect on the efficacy of NRT, its ascertainment is a 'must do' criterion.

- *For those who have consulted in the last 12 months the records show that, at least annually, motivated patients who smoke more than 10 cigarettes a day have been recommended to use nicotine replacement therapy*

Eight weeks' treatment with NRT should be recommended for motivated smokers who consume more than 10 cigarettes daily since extended courses of NRT are no more effective (Silagy *et al.*, 1997). The undisputed efficacy of NRT demands that recommending its use appropriately is a 'must do' criterion. Although NRT cannot be issued on an NHS prescription in the UK, GPs can recommend its use or supply it by private prescription. Virtually all NRT studies have involved prescription of NRT accompanied by advice or support from a clinician, and it is unlikely that NRT will otherwise exert any beneficial effect. A follow-up appointment for NRT users is, therefore, essential.

- *The records show that pregnant smokers have had smoking cessation discussed with them and those who are motivated to stop are offered a follow-up appointment*

Advice to stop smoking from doctors, nurses and midwives is effective in helping pregnant smokers to stop (Dolan-Mullen *et al.*, 1994; Lumley, 1995). As there is clear evidence that advice is effective when given to pregnant women, the recording of such advice is a 'must do' criterion. It should be explained to pregnant women that smoking is associated with intrauterine growth retardation and low birth-weight babies (Dolan-Mullen *et al.*, 1994). Midwives and GPs are ideally placed to repeatedly raise the topic of smoking at antenatal appointments.

Undertaking the audit

Clinicians in your practice must meet and decide where to start. You may wish to begin by completing the form in Chapter 3, Box 3.2, before writing your audit plan. You will need to generate a list of patients for inclusion in the audit. Most practices will have smoking status recorded for at least some patients, as this was necessary to claim health promotion payments under the recently terminated 'banding scheme' (NHS Management Executive, 1993). It may be possible, therefore, to compile a list of smokers who have consulted in the past 12 months using the same reporting tools that you used to provide health promotion data. However, you will only be able to use this retrospective approach for identifying smokers if your definitions for smoking behaviour, at the time you collected the data, were the same as ours (Box 7.2).

If differences exist, you should use our definitions (Box 7.2) to collect the smokers' names prospectively. You will need to specify a time period during which smokers are to be identified and decide which members of the primary health care team are to participate in compiling a list of smokers. Next, smokers who attend participating members of the primary health care team will have their details recorded on an encounter sheet. By doing this you will identify a cohort of patients for inclusion in the audit and data collection can begin. If a large number of smokers is identified, you may need to sample (see Chapter 3). Examples of data collection forms are included at the end of the chapter. Figure 7.2 is a form for recording audit data on individual smokers and Figure 7.3 is for recording data on a maximum of 10 smokers. Once the first data collection phase is complete, the participants involved in the audit need to meet and agree necessary changes and plan for the second data collection phase.

Data collection form **Smoking cessation protocol**

Name	
DOB	
Age	
Id No.	

Criterion 1

Smoking status recorded   y☐   n☐   dk☐
in last twelve months

Quantity recorded   y☐   n☐   dk☐

Criterion 2

Smoking cessation   y☐   n☐   dk☐
discussed

Follow-up offered/   y☐   n☐   dk☐
taken place

Criterion 3

Motivation to stop   y☐   n☐   dk☐
assessed

Criterion 4

Smoking > 10/day   y☐   n☐   dk☐

Motivation to stop   y☐   n☐   dk☐

Offered NRT   y☐   n☐   dk☐

Criterion 5

Pregnant smokers   y☐   n☐   nk☐

Smoking cessation   y☐   n☐   nk☐
discussed

Follow-up offered/   y☐   n☐   nk☐
taken place

Figure 7.2 Data collection form for individual patient

Data collection form

Practice code

✓ = Yes, ✗ = No, O = DK

Smoking cessation protocol

Patient	Age	Sex	Smoking status checked in last 12 months	Quantity smoked recorded	Advice given	Motivation assessed	Offered follow-up	NRT offered if motivated and >10 per day	Pregnant smokers	
									Advice given	Follow-up offered/taken place

Figure 7.3 Data collection form: 10 patients per form

Key points

- Smoking continues to be associated with considerable morbidity and mortality and consequent health care costs.

- GPs and other members of the primary health care team can play a key role in influencing patients to stop smoking through opportunistic intervention as patients consult.

- As a first step, the motivation of patients towards stopping smoking must be ascertained.

- For motivated patients who smoke more than 10 cigarettes daily, an 8 week course of nicotine replacement therapy should be recommended.

- GPs and other members of the primary health care team must be prepared to discuss smoking cessation repeatedly with smokers.

References

Ashenden, R., Silagy, C. and Weller, D. (1997) A systematic review of the effectiveness of promoting lifestyle change in general practice. *Fam. Pract.* **14**: 160–176.

Coleman, T. and Wilson, A. (1996) Anti-smoking advice in general practice consultations: GPs' attitudes, reported practice and perceived problems. *Br. J. Gen. Pract.* **46**: 87–91.

Di Clemente, C.C., Prochaska, J.O., Fairhurst, S.K. *et al.* (1991). The process of smoking cessation: an analysis of precontemplation, contemplation and preparation stages of change. *J. Consult. Clin. Psychol.* **59**: 295–304.

Dolan-Mullen, P., Ramirez, G. and Groff, J.Y. (1994) A meta-analysis of randomized trials of prenatal smoking cessation interventions. *Am. J. Obstet. Gynecol.* **171** (5): 1328–1334.

Doll, R. and Peto, R. (1976) Mortality in relation to smoking: 20 years' observation on male British doctors. *BMJ* **2**: 1525–1530.

Fiore, M.C., Bailey, W.C., Cohen, S.J. *et al.* (1996) Smoking Cessation. Clinical Practice Guideline No. 18. Rockville, MD: US Department of Health and Human Services, Public Health Service/Agency for Health Care Policy and Research (AHCPR Publication No. 96-0692).

Health Education Authority (1991) *The Smoking Epidemic: counting the cost.* London, HEA.

Jackson, P.H., Stapleton, J.A., Russell, M.A.H. and Merriman, R.J. (1986) Predictors of outcome in a GP intervention against smoking. *Prevent. Med.* **15**: 244–253.

Jamrozik, K., Vessey, M., Fowler, G. *et al.* (1984). Controlled trial of three different anti-smoking interventions in general practice. *BMJ* **288**: 1499–1503.

Kottke, T.E., Battista, R.N., De Friese, G.H. and Brekke, M.L. (1988) Attributes of successful smoking interventions in medical practice: a meta-analysis of 39 controlled trials. *JAMA* **259**: 2883–2889.

Lumley, J. (1995) Advice as a strategy for reducing smoking in pregnancy. In *Pregnancy and Child Birth Module* (Eds Enkin, M.W., Keirse, M.J.N.C., Refrew, M.J. and Neilson, J.P.), Cochrane Pregnancy and Childbirth 'Database': Review no. 03394.1995, issue 2. Oxford: Update Software.

Marlatt, G.A., Curry, S. and Gordon, R. (1988) A longitudinal analysis of unaided smoking cessation. *J. Consult. Clin. Psychol.* **56**: 715–770.

Marsh, A. and Matheson, J. (1983) *Smoking Attitudes and Behaviour*, pp. 118–126. London: HMSO.

NHS Management Executive (1993) GP contract health promotion package: amendments to the statement of fees and allowances. FHSL (93) 25. London: Department of Health.

Office of Population Censuses and Surveys (1994) *General Household Survey 1992* (Series GHS, No. 23, GB, Age 16+). London: HMSO.

Russell, M.A.H., Merriman, R., Stapleton, J. and Taylor, W. (1983) Effect of nicotine chewing gum as an adjunct to GPs' advice against smoking. *BMJ* **287**: 1782–1783.

Russell, M.A.H., Wilson, C., Taylor, C. and Baker, C.B. (1979) Effect of GPs' advice against smoking. *BMJ* **2**: 231–235.

Silagy, C. and Ketteridge, S. (1996) The effectiveness of physician advice to aid smoking cessation. In *Tobacco Addiction Module* (Eds Lancaster, T. and Silagy, C.), Cochrane Database of Systematic Reviews, The Cochrane Collaboration: issue 1 (updated quarterly). Oxford: Update Software.

Silagy, C., Mant, D., Fowler, G. and Lancaster, T. (1997) The effect of nicotine replacement therapy on smoking cessation. In *Tobacco Addiction Module* (Eds Lancaster, T., Silagy, C. and Fullerton, D.), Cochrane Database of Systematic Reviews, The Cochrane Collaboration: issue 2 (updated quarterly). Oxford: Update Software.

Silagy, C., Muir, J., Coulter, A., *et al.* (1992) Lifestyle advice in general practice: rates recalled by patients. *BMJ* **305**: 871–874.

Slama, K., Karsenty, S. and Hirsch, A. (1995) Effectiveness of minimal intervention by GPs with their smoking patients: a randomized, controlled trial in France. *Tobacco Control* **4**: 162–169.

Williams, S.J. and Calnan, M. (1994) Perspectives on prevention: the views of GPs. *Sociology of Health and Illness* **16**: 372–395.

Yudkin, P.L., Jones, L., Lancaster, T. *et al.* (1996) Which smokers are helped to give up smoking using transdermal nicotine patches? Results from a randomized double-blind, placebo-controlled trial. *Br. J. Gen. Pract.* **46**: 145–148.

8

Improving mental health: a protocol for an audit of the care of patients with depression

Introduction

Depression is common and its recognition and management in primary care are often less than ideal. Up to 50 per cent of patients consulting their GP will have some depressive symptoms (Freeling and Tylee, 1992), of whom around 5 per cent will have major depression (Vazquez-Barquero et al., 1987). Following diagnosis, most depressed adult patients can readily be managed in general practice with antidepressant medication and/or cognitive therapy. Both have been shown to be effective treatments, although prescribed medication is often given in inadequate doses for too short a period of time (Freeling et al., 1985; Donoghue and Tylee, 1996).

In this chapter we describe the development of an audit protocol which should assist practices to improve their management of patients with depression.

Scope

The protocol is for primary health care teams and does not consider the management of patients after referral to specialist services. Patients with major depression (sometimes referred to as unipolar depression) are included, and by definition episodes of major depression last at least 2 weeks. Bipolar disorders, postnatal and recurrent depression are excluded. The use of secondary treatments such as monoamine oxidase inhibitors (MAOI), electroconvulsive therapy (ECT) and lithium is also excluded. The protocol relates to adult patients over the age of 18 years.

The protocol also excludes the detection of depression, although it is well established that a high proportion of depressed patients attending GPs do not have their depression diagnosed (Skuse and Williams, 1994; Freeling et al., 1985).

The key elements of care relating to diagnosis, management and follow-up of patients with depression were identified from a systematic review (NHS Centre for Reviews and Dissemination, 1993), consensus guidelines (Paykel and Priest, 1992; Clinical Resource and Audit Group, 1993) and an evidence-based guideline (US Department of Health and Human Services, 1993). To develop the criteria, a focused literature search was undertaken.

Audit criteria and their justification

'Must do' criteria

The following criteria have been categorized as 'must do' (see Box 8.1).

Box 8.1   Criteria for the management of depression

'Must do' criteria
- The records show that the diagnosis is correct.
- The records show that at diagnosis the patient has been assessed for risk of suicide.
- Patients with 'major depression' are treated with antidepressants and/or cognitive therapy.
- Antidepressants must be prescribed in therapeutic doses.

'Should do' criteria
- Drug treatment should be continued for at least 4 months after the symptoms of depression have resolved.
- After commencement of treatment the patient should be reviewed within 3 weeks to monitor response to treatment and compliance; and to reassess suicide risk.
- Patients who have responded fully in the acute phase of treatment are seen at least once every month during the maintenance of treatment.

- *The records show that the diagnosis of depression is correct*

The literature review indicated that the key to diagnosing and managing patients with depression is the recognition of particular 'core' symptoms and/or signs which must have been present for at least 2 weeks. We recommend use of the International Statistical Classification on Mental and Behavioural disorders (ICD-10) (World Health Organisation, 1992) which is the most commonly used classification in this country (see Box 8.2). The other classification in use is the DSM – IV (American Psychiatric Association, 1994).

Box. 8.2   Symptoms and signs required for the diagnosis of depression (ICD-10)
- Low or sad mood.
- Loss of interest or pleasure.
- Associated symptoms are frequently present:
     disturbed sleep;
     guilt or low self-worth;
     fatigue or loss of energy;
     poor concentration;
     disturbed appetite;
     suicidal thoughts or acts.
- Movements and speech may be slowed, but patient may also appear agitated.
- Symptoms of anxiety or nervousness are frequently also present.

The classification systems are important because they enable a distinction to be made between those patients who have transient mood disturbance and who do not benefit from anti-depressant treatment and those who have a clinical disorder consisting of a constellation of symptoms and signs who do benefit from treatment. The prescription of antidepressant medication to patients who are sad rather than clinically depressed is not justifiable.

In summary, this criterion was classified as 'must do' because there is evidence of misdiagnosis. Some cases are not detected, and other patients receive treatment unnecessarily. Randomized controlled trial evidence of the effectiveness of treatment relates to patients who meet the established diagnostic classifications.

- *The records show that at diagnosis the patient has been assessed for risk of suicide*

Suicide is the most dramatic consequence of depression. A target was set in the *Health of the Nation* strategy for reducing the suicide rate by at least 15 per cent by the year 2000, from 11.1 to no more than 9.4 per 100 000 of the population (Department of Health, 1992). Unfortunately, the benefits of routine evaluation of suicide risk in primary care have not been rigorously assessed, although recent studies do provide limited evidence that the rate of suicide may be reduced through training GPs to assess suicide risk (Rutz *et al.*, 1992a,b). Although it is difficult to evaluate the effects of interventions to reduce suicides amongst unselected depressed patients, small studies involving patients who had previously attempted suicide have been undertaken, but firm conclusions must await the findings of a systematic review (Hawton *et al.*, 1997).

Indirect evidence that supports a policy of assessing suicide risk can be found in studies that show that optimal pharmacotherapy (Shou and Weeke, 1988) and routine psychiatric consultation after attempted suicide (Greer and Bagley, 1971) both reduce suicides. Furthermore, most depressed patients who commit suicide are not taking antidepressants immediately before death (Isacsson *et al.*, 1994). Although there is a clear link between depression and suicide, accurate prediction of which patients will attempt suicide is nevertheless difficult in general practice (Lin *et al.*, 1989). The risk factors that have been related to suicide include general medical illness, a personal or family history of substance abuse, history of a prior suicide attempt, the presence of psychotic symptoms and the time of year (spring and early summer). Young males, immigrants (especially females), the divorced and those in social class V have an increased risk of suicide.

In summary, this criterion was classified as 'must do' because suicide is the most important negative outcome caused by depression. Although there is no direct RCT evidence that risk assessment is effective, evidence from a controlled trial and small randomized trials involving patients in a high risk group do provide support for this approach. Consequently, a randomized trial in which the risk of suicide of the control group of patients was not assessed would be un-likely to gain ethical approval.

- *Patients with 'major depression' are treated with antidepressants and/or cognitive therapy*

Antidepressants have been shown to be effective treatments in general practice for patients with depressive disorders that comply with the criteria for major depressive illness (Thompson and Thompson, 1989; Paykel *et al.*, 1988). Tricyclic antidepressants (TCAs) and selective serotonin reuptake inhibitors (SSRIs) are the two main groups of antidepressant drugs in common use (NHS Centre for Reviews and Dissemination, 1993).

Opinions differ on the choice of antidepressant. Although SSRIs may be associated with a lower proportion of patients stopping treatment (Anderson and Tomenson, 1995; Martin *et al.*, 1997), they may be more expensive (NHS Centre for Reviews and Dissemination, 1993). The most commonly recommended approach is to tailor the choice of drug to the individual patient, taking into account factors such as risk of suicide (Henry *et al.*, 1995), side-effects, prior response to medication, concurrent illnesses, concurrent use of other medications and likelihood of compliance (US Department of Health and Human Services, 1993; MeRec Bulletin, 1995).

Preferred psychotherapeutic approaches are those shown to benefit patients in research trials, such as interpersonal, cognitive, behavioural and brief dynamic therapies. RCTs of psychotherapy have been limited to patients with less severe forms of major depression. Therefore, patients with mild to moderate depression may be treated with this option but those with severe depression must be treated with medication with or without psychotherapy (US Department of Health and Human Services, 1993).

In summary, this criterion was classified as 'must do' because research evidence confirms the beneficial impact on outcome of antidepressants and/or cognitive therapy.

- *Antidepressants must be prescribed in therapeutic doses*

Despite advice contained in widely available guidelines, it is common in general practice for depressed patients to be prescribed a sub-therapeutic dose of an antidepressant (Donohughe *et al.*, 1996). Several placebo-controlled studies have shown that low doses of antidepressants are ineffective (Thompson and Thompson, 1989; Blaski *et al.*, 1971). There was no evidence in these studies that the therapeutic dose of 150 mg of amitriptyline produced more side-effects than a sub-therapeutic dose of 75 mg per day. A recent primary care study in Scotland also confirmed that antidepressants are still commonly prescribed for inadequate durations and in low doses (MacDonald *et al.*, 1996). Furthermore, the risk of suicide among patients with psychiatric disorder has been found to decrease with optimal pharmacotherapy (Shou and Weeke, 1988; Barraclough, 1972).

Thus, this criterion was classified as 'must do' because there is evidence that patients often receive low doses of antidepressant which are not therapeutically effective.

'Should do' criteria

The following criteria have been categorized as 'should do' (see Box 8.1).

- *Drug treatment should be continued for at least 4 months after the symptoms of depression have resolved*

Depression is a chronic and often recurrent illness. In a 5 year prospective study of the natural history of major depression, 28 per cent of patients reported recurrence of symptoms within 1 year and 62 per cent within 5 years (Keller *et al.*, 1992). Continuation of treatment is undertaken to decrease the likelihood of relapse. Early discontinuation of treatment has been shown to be followed by a 25 per cent relapse rate within 2 months. Patients more likely to relapse include those with a history of previous episodes of depression, severe illness, residual symptoms after treatment and a lack of social support. RCTs involving outpatients have shown that continued treatment with antidepressants for several months after symptoms have resolved leads to a significantly reduced rate of relapse and recurrence (NHS Centre for Reviews and Dissemination, 1993). However, studies of the effectiveness of longer-term treatment in general practice are required. Although some general practice patients are likely to need treatment for several months, it is not clear whether this is necessary for all.

In summary, this criterion was classified as 'should do' because, although there is good evidence that treatment continued for 4 months after the resolution of symtoms improves long-term outcome, the evidence is limited to patients attending a hospital outpatient department.

- *After commencement of treatment patients should be reviewed within 3 weeks to monitor response to treatment and compliance and to reassess suicide risk*

At least 2–4 weeks of antidepressant treatment with serum levels within the therapeutic range are required before a patient can be regarded as not responding. If the patient has not responded by 6 weeks, the dose or drug may be changed, or serum drug levels checked (US Department of Health and Human Services, 1993).

In studies of compliance with antidepressants, between 20 per cent (Thompson *et al.*, 1982) and 59 per cent (Johnson, 1973) of patients discontinued treatment within 3 weeks. Therefore, it is important to review patients to check compliance and offer advice about treatment. Since there are no RCTs to show if this has any impact on outcome, this criterion was classified as 'should do'.

• Patients who have responded fully in the acute phase of treatment are seen at least once every month during the maintenance of treatment

There are no RCTs to show if this has any direct impact on outcome. This criterion was based on the consensus that emerged during peer review of the protocol, and was supported by guidelines (US Department of Health and Human Services, 1993) that it was good clinical practice to monitor patients at intervals during the continuation phase of treatment. In addition, if there is significant continuation or reappearance of symptoms, referral to a psychiatrist must be considered. On the other hand, some patients are continued on medication long after it could have been withdrawn (Duncan and Campbell, 1988). Therefore, patients should be reviewed to check that treatment is still appropriate.

Undertaking the audit

Identification of patients

If you use a computerized patient record, it is a simple matter to identify all patients currently attending with depression and undertake a retrospective first-stage data collection (see Chapter 3). If not, you will need to identify and compile a list of patients with depression as they attend for consultations. The doctors should be provided with a standard form for recording depressed patients – an encounter form. If you have a large number of patients with depression, you can select a random sample (see Chapter 3).

Data collection

In this audit data are collected from the records of patients with depression. The method is described in Chapter 3. In outline, a member of the practice (e.g. GP, practice nurse) is appointed to co-ordinate the audit. The records of patients are extracted from the filing system and are entered on data collection forms (see Figures 8.1 and 8.2). Data analysis is undertaken in the usual way.

When considering implementing changes, practices should first identify the reasons for failing to comply with the criteria. There may be many different reasons, for example reticence regarding asking about suicide risk, pressure on appointments, or lack of adequate secondary care services such as cognitive therapy. The practice should then plan practical strategies to address these problems prior to the second data collection phase.

Data collection form   **Depression protocol**

Patient code No.			Current medical treatment	
DOB			Tricyclics	
Sex	M	F	SSRI	
Date of diagnosis			Other	
			Cognitive therapy	
			Referred to psychiatrist or mental health team	

Criterion 1
Diagnosis of depression correct?   y☐   n☐   nk☐

Criterion 2
The records show that at diagnosis the patient has been assessed for risk of suicide?   y☐   n☐   nk☐

Patient at risk   y☐   n☐   nk☐

If suicide risk identified, action taken: *referred as:*
in-patient ☐
out-patient ☐
drug treatment ☐
none ☐
other ☐
(specify _____)

Criterion 3
Patient has 'major depression'   y☐   n☐   nk☐

If yes, treated with:
antidepressants ☐
cognitive therapy ☐
other ☐
n/k ☐

Criterion 4
Antidepressants prescribed in therapeutic doses?   y☐   n☐   nk☐

Criterion 5
Symptoms of depression resolved?   y☐   n☐   nk☐

If treatment commenced 4 or more months ago, treatment continued for 4 months?   y☐   n☐

If treatment commenced less than 4 months ago, patient continues to receive treatment?   y☐   n☐

If treatment discontinued within 4 months, state why.   ———

Criterion 6
If treatment started, patient reviewed within 3 weeks?   y☐   n☐   nk☐

Risk of suicide reassessed?   y☐   n☐   nk☐

Criterion 7
Reviewed every month during treatment?   y☐   n☐   nk☐

Figure 8.1 Data collection form for individual patient

Data collection form

Depression protocol

Must do ✓ = Yes **x** = No n = not known blank = not applicable

Should do

Background data

Pat. code No.	DOB	Sex	Treatment T- Trcyclics S-SSRI O-other C-cognitive therapy R-refer

1 Diagnosis correct

2 Records show suicide risk assessed? — At risk

If yes, action taken: Referred | Drug treatment | None | Other specify

3 Patient has major depression

If yes, treated with: Anti-depressants | Cognitive therapy | Other | Not known

4 Anti-depressants prescribed in therapeutic doses?

Name medication and total daily dose (mg)

5 Episode for depression resolved

If treatment commenced 4 or more months ago, treatment continued for 4 months?

If treatment commenced less than 4 months ago, patient continued to receive treatment?

If treatment discontinued within 4 months state why

6 If treatment started, patient reviewed within 3 weeks?

Risk of suicide assessed?

7 Reviewed every month during treatment?

TOTALS

Figure 8.2 Data collection form: 10 patients per form

Key points

- Depression is a common condition which causes much morbidity and some mortality through increased risk of suicide.

- The vast majority of patients with depression can be treated by GPs without referral to a psychiatrist.

- There is overwhelming evidence that many GPs: (1) do not recognize depression when the patient first presents; and/or (2) prescribe anti-depressants in inadequate doses for too short a period.

- Consequently, an audit of the management of patients with depression should assist GPs to improve the quality of care.

References

American Psychiatric Association (1994) *Diagnostic and Statistical Manual of Mental Disorders*, 4th Edn. Washington, DC: APA.

Anderson, I.M. and Tomenson, B.M. (1995) Treatment discontinuation with selective serotonin reuptake inhibitors compared with tricyclic antidepressants: a meta-analysis. *BMJ* **310**: 1433–1438.

Barraclough, B. (1972) Suicide prevention, recurrent affective disorder and lithium. *Br. J. Psychiat.* **121**: 391–392.

Blashki, T.G., Mowbray, R. and Davies, B. (1971) Controlled trial of amitriptyline in general practice. *BMJ* **1**: 133–138.

Clinical Resourse and Audit Group (1993) Depressive illness: a critical review of current practice and the way ahead. Consensus statement. The Scottish Office: National Health Service in Scotland.

Department of Health (1992) *The Health of the Nation: a strategy for health in England*. London: HMSO.

Donohughe, J.M. and Tylee, A. (1996) The treatment of depression: prescribing patterns of antidepressants in primary care in the UK. *Br. J. Psychiat.* **168**: 164–168.

Duncan, A.J. and Campbell, A.J. (1988) Antidepressant drugs in the elderly: are the indications as long term as the treatment? *BMJ* **296**: 1230–1232.

Freeling, P., Rao, B.M., Paykel, E.S. *et al.* (1985) Unrecognised depression in general practice. *BMJ* **290**: 1880–1883.

Freeling, P. and Tylee, A. (1992) Depression in general practice. In *Handbook of Affective Disorders*, 2nd Ed (Ed. Paykel, E.S.). Edinburgh: Churchill Livingstone.

Greer, S. and Bagley, C. (1971) Effect of psychiatric intervention in attempted suicide: a controlled study. *BMJ* **1**: 310–312.

Hawton, K., Arensman, E. and Townsend, E. (1997) Systematic review of treatment studies of patients who have attempted suicide (protocol), Cochrane Library: issue 3. Oxford: Update Software.

Henry, J.A., Alexander, C.A. and Sener, E.K. (1995) Relative mortality from overdose of antidepressant. *BMJ* **310**: 221–224.

Johnson, D.A.W. (1973) Treatment of depression in general practice. *BMJ* **2**: 18–20.

Isacsson, G., Holmgren, P., Wasserman, D. and Beryman, U. (1994) Use of antidepressants among people committing suicide in Sweden. *BMJ* **308**: 506–509.

Keller, M.B., Lavori, P.W., Mueller, T.I. *et al.* (1992) Time to recovery, chronicity and levels of psychopathology in major depression: a 5 year prospective follow-up of 431 subjects. *Arch. Gen. Psychiat.* **49**: 809–816.

Lin, E.H.B., von Korff, M. and Wagner, E.H. (1989) Identifying suicide potential in primary care. *J. Gen. Int. Med.* **4**: 1–6.

MacDonald, T.M., McMahon, A.D., Reid, I.C., (1996) Antidepressant drug care in primary care: a record linkage study in Tayside, Scotland. *BMJ* **313**: 860–861.

Martin, R.M., Hilton, S.R., Kerry, S.M. and Richards, N.M. (1997) General practitioners' perceptions of the tolerability of antidepressant drugs: a comparison of selective serotonin reuptake inhibitors and tricyclic antidepressants. *BMJ* **314**: 646–651.

MeReC Bulletin (1995) Volume 6 (1). Liverpool: Medicines Resource Centre.

NHS Centre for Reviews and Dissemination (1993). Effective health care: the treatment of depression in primary care (Bulletin No. 5). Leeds: University of Leeds.

Paykel, E.S., Hollyman, J.A., Freeling, P. and Sedwick, P. (1988) Predictors of therapeutic benefit from amitriptyline in mild depression: a general practice placebo-controlled trial. *J. Affective Disord.* **14**: 83–95.

Paykel, E.S. and Priest, R.G. (1992) Recognition and management of depression in general practice: consensus statement. *BMJ* **305**: 1198–1202.

Rutz, W., Carlsson, P., von Knorring, L. and Walinder, J. (1992a) Cost–benefit analysis of an educational programme for general practitioners by the Swedish Committee for the Prevention and Treatment of Depression. *Acta Psychiatr. Scand.* **85**: 457–464.

Rutz, W., von Knorring, L. and Walinder, J. (1992b) Long-term effects of an educational program for general practitioners given by the Swedish Committee for the Prevention and Treatment of Depression. *Acta Psychiatr. Scand.* **85**: 83–88.

Shou, M. and Weeke, A. (1988) Did manic-depressive patients who committed suicide receive prophylactic or continuation treatment at the time? *Br. J. Psychiat.* **153**: 324–327.

Skuse, D. and Williams, P. (1984) Screening for psychiatric disorder in general practice. *J. Psychol. Med.* **14**: 365–377.

Thomson, J., Rankin, H., Ashcroft, G.W. *et al.* (1982) The treatment of depression in general practice: a comparison of L-tryptophan, amitriptyline, and a combination of L-tryptophan and amitriptyline with placebo. *J. Psychol. Med.* **12**: 741–751.

Thomson, C. and Thomson, C.M. (1989) The prescribing of antidepressants in general practice II: A placebo-controlled trial of low-dose dothiepin. *Human Psychopharmacol.* **4**: 191–204.

US Department of Health and Human Services (1993) *Clinical Practice Guideline Number 5. Depression in Primary Care, Volumes 1 and 2. Treatment of Major Depression.* Rockville: AHCPR Publications.

Vasquez-Barquero, J., Diez-Manrique, J.F., Pena, C. *et al.* (1987) A community mental health survey in Cantabria: a general description of morbidity. *J. Psychol. Med.* **17**: 227–241.

World Health Organisation (1992) International Statistical Classification of Mental and Behavioural Disorders, 10th revision. Geneva: WHO.

Appendix 1 Other available Lilly Centre audit protocols: lists of 'must do' criteria

This appendix contains the 'must do' criteria from the other audit protocols developed to date by the Eli Lilly National Clinical Audit Centre. These protocols are available from your local MAAG or can be ordered through:

Eli Lilly National Clinical Audit Centre,
Department of General Practice and Primary Health Care,
Leicester University,
Leicester General Hospital,
Gwendolen Road,
Leicester LE5 4PW, UK

Telephone: (0116) 258 4873
Fax: (0116) 258 4982
E-mail: clinaudit@le.ac.uk

Other protocols available:

- Monitoring asthma
- Benzodiazepines: long-term users
- Benzodiazepines: new prescriptions
- Patient's Charter protocols: Home visits and Repeat prescription systems
- Management of angina in general practice
- Gout
- Monitoring lithium treatment
- Management of hypertension in primary practice
- Heart failure
- Osteoporosis

Monitoring asthma
'Must do' criteria

1. Patients who have been diagnosed as asthmatic will be recorded in the practice asthma register.

2. The diagnosis of asthma has been confirmed (i.e. a patient recorded as asthmatic must have been shown to definitely have asthma).

3. The records show that, at least annually, an assessment is made of the level of control of asthma by assessment of nocturnal and daytime symptoms and limitations on daily activities.

4. The records show that, at least annually, the daily dose of bronchodilator has been checked and that those patients who require more than one dose daily are also receiving prophylactic medication.

5. The records show that the patient's smoking habits are recorded at least annually, and for children, the smoking habits of adults in the household are recorded and advice given.

6. The records show that, at least annually, the inhaler technique has been checked.

7. The records show that, at least annually, each asthmatic patient and/or their carer(s) has received education about:
   (i) the recognition of danger signs of an asthma attack; and
   (ii) the importance of seeking medical help early during an attack.

(Developed 1994)

Benzodiazepines: long-term users
'Must do' criteria

1. All patients on long-term benzodiazepines must be recorded on a specific register or a computerized repeat prescribing system.

2. The records must show that long-term users of benzodiazepines have been assessed on their suitability for withdrawal.

3. Patients assessed suitable for withdrawal must be told about dependency, withdrawal recommended and this recorded in their notes.

4. Patients who are unsuitable for withdrawal or not ready to withdraw must continue to receive their medication.

5. Withdrawal from benzodiazepines must be a phased reduction in the drug over a period of no less than 6 weeks.

6. The records must show that patients undertaking withdrawal have received information about symptoms to expect and coping strategies.

7. The records must show that patients failing to withdraw or not ready to withdraw are reviewed at least annually.

(Developed 1994)

Benzodiazepines: new prescriptions
'Must do' criteria

1. The records must show that a patient receiving a new prescription for a benzodiazepine has been advised on non-drug therapies for anxiety or insomnia.

2. New benzodiazepine prescriptions must be reserved for short-term relief of severe anxiety or insomnia.

3. If a benzodiazepine is prescribed, the records show that the patient has been advised on the potential for dependency.

(Developed 1995)

Patient's Charter protocols
'Must do' criteria: Home visits

1. There must be a written practice policy for responding to requests for home visits (including emergency, urgent and non-urgent visits).

2. Each patient who requests an urgent or non-urgent home visit must either:
   (i) have a visit agreed; or
   (ii) talk directly to a GP immediately.

3. Emergency visits must be carried out immediately.

4. Urgent visits must be carried out within 2 hours.

5. When a request for a non-urgent visit is accepted, the patient must be given an approximate visit time. If the GP is delayed, the patient must be informed of the new expected visit time.

(Developed 1994)

'Must do' criteria: Repeat prescription systems

1. Patients' requests for repeat prescriptions must be processed within 24 hours, excluding weekends and bank holidays.

2. Patients receiving repeat prescriptions must have a card/record sheet with which to request their prescriptions, which includes:
   - the name of each drug;
   - the dose of each drug;
   - the quantity of each drug prescribed.
   - the date of the last supply for each drug;

- the number of repeats allowed, and/or the next review date for each drug.

3. For patients receiving repeat prescriptions, the medical records must contain a repeat prescribing card, computer print-out or drug list which indicates:
   - the name of each drug;
   - the dose of each drug;
   - the quantity of all drugs prescribed;
   - the date of the last supply for each drug;
   - the number of repeats allowed and/or the next review date for each drug.

4. The patient-held card or record sheet, the medical record card and the computer system (if there is one) must all contain the same information about the medication.

(Developed 1994)

Management of angina in general practice
'Must do' criteria

1. The records show that the diagnosis of angina is based on: (a) characteristic symptoms of angina or (b) suggestive symptoms of angina supported by positive investigations.

2. The records show that at diagnosis the blood pressure has been recorded, the patient examined for signs of anaemia, and a cardiac examination has been carried out.

3. The records show that the patient is on daily aspirin unless contraindicated.

4. The records show that, at least annually, there has been an assessment of smoking habit, and advice given to smokers.

5. The records show that at diagnosis the patient's blood lipids have been checked.

6. The records show that, at least annually, the blood pressure has been checked and is within normal limits.

7. The records show that there is an annual assessment of symptoms.

(Developed 1995)

Gout
'Must do' criteria

1. The diagnosis of gout is correct.

2. The records show that in the absence of contraindications, acute attacks of gout are treated with non-steroidal anti-inflammatory medication.

3. The records show that risk factors (alcohol intake, obesity and diuretics) have been recorded and appropriate advice given.

4. Antihyperuricaemic therapy has only been used after a second attack of gout (and not for symptomless hyperuricaemia).

(Developed 1995)

Monitoring lithium treatment
'Must do' criteria

1. Patients who are receiving lithium treatment must be recorded in a practice lithium register.

2. The records show that the serum lithium concentration has been checked on at least four occasions in the last 12 months at 3 monthly intervals.

3. The records show that the lithium concentration is within the therapeutic range of 0.4–0.8 mmol/l.

4. The records show that, at least annually, the patient has been assessed for clinical evidence of thyroid disease including goitre.

(Developed 1995)

Management of hypertension in primary practice
'Must do' criteria

1. Patients who have been diagnosed as hypertensive have been recorded in a practice hypertension register.

2. The records show that, in patients without target organ damage, the blood pressure has been measured at least twice on each of at least three separate occasions prior to commencement of drug therapy.

3. The records show that, at diagnosis, the following symptoms and signs of target organ damage have been sought: retinopathy, left ventricular hypertrophy, angina, stroke, heart failure, peripheral vascular disease and renal disease.

4. The records show that an assessment has been made of the risk factors for cardiovascular and cerebrovascular disease and that, if necessary, appropriate advice and treatment has been given. Risk factors involved are: smoking habit, body mass index, diabetes mellitus, serum cholesterol (if additional risk factors present), excessive alcohol intake, physical inactivity and family history of premature coronary artery disease.

5. The records show that the mean pretreatment blood pressure level was at least a diastolic of 95 mmHg or greater and/or a systolic of 160 mmHg or greater, or a diastolic of 90–95 mmHg in the presence of other cardiovascular risk factors and/or target organ damage.

6. The records show that the patient has been reviewed at regular intervals not exceeding 6 months.

7. The records show that the hypertension is well controlled, the average of the last three recorded diastolic blood pressure readings being 90 mmHg (diastolic) or below, and 160 mmHg (systolic) or below.

8. The records show that a patient with refractory hypertension and/or suspected secondary hypertension has been referred for specialist advice.

(Developed 1995)

Heart failure
'Must do' criteria

1. The records show that the clinical diagnosis of heart failure is based on characteristic symptoms of heart failure and confirmed by (i) a chest X-ray, and/or (ii) echocardiogram.

2. A patient suspected of having heart failure must have an echocardiogram if he/she has a murmur on clinical examination.

3. The records show that patients diagnosed as having heart failure have been commenced on a diuretic.

4. The records show that patients with left ventricular systolic dysfunction have been commenced on an angiotensin converting enzyme inhibitor unless there are contraindications.

5. The records show that the blood pressure has been recorded annually and is in the normal range.

6. The records show that patients with heart failure are commenced on digoxin if:
   (i) they remain symptomatic despite optimal management with an ACE inhibitor and diuretics; or
   (ii) symptomatic patients are unable to tolerate ACE inhibitors;
   (iii) the patient is in atrial fibrillation.

(Developed 1998)

If the answer to any of the above questions is 'no', amend/correct before proceeding any further.

2. Planning phase

- Has the relevant literature been reviewed adequately?
- Have explicit criteria been identified?
- Are the criteria:
  - relevant?
  - measurable?
  - evidence-based?
  - prioritized?
- Have explicit standards been set for all criteria?
- Are the proposed data collection methods:
  - clearly described?
  - appropriate for the task?
- Are the data to be collected relevant to the aims of the audit?
- Have all data collection forms been prepared?
- Is there a procedure for monitoring completeness of data collection?
- Is the proposed audit population/sample/number of events:
  - adequate?
  - representative?
- Is the proposed method of analysis:
  - clearly stated?
  - appropriate?
- If sampling, does the analysis include 95% C.I.s?
- Have all participants been fully briefed on aims, methodology and their expected role?

3. Operational phase

First data collection

- Have all the agreed data been collected and/or is the response rate adequate?
- Have the results been compared directly with the standards set for each agreed criterion in turn?
- Are the expected standards still realistic?
- Have the results been:
  - distributed to all participants?
  - discussed with all participants?
- Have required changes been:
  - identified?
  - agreed for implementation?
- Are these changes realistic?
- Has a realistic time interval been agreed between the first and second data collection phases?

Second data collection

- Have all the agreed data been collected and/or is the response rate adequate?
- For each agreed criterion in turn, have the results been compared directly with:
  - the standards set?
  - the results of the first data collection?
- Have the results been:
  - distributed to all participants?
  - discussed with all participants?
- If expected changes have not been made, have credible and acceptable reasons been identified?
- Have areas requiring further change been identified?
- Has the need for a further audit cycle been considered?

4. Review and report phase

- Is the audit reported in a systematic way?
- Is the report written in clear and understandable language?
- Does the report contain a succinct summary of the key issues and conclusions?
- Does the report contain a clear description of the impact of the audit, i.e. the extent of improvements for patients, professionals or the service?
- Is there an adequate list of references?

Index

Note: page references in **bold** indicate tables or figures; these pages may also contain textual references